Narcissism and Codependency

Learn How to Deal with a Narcissistic Personality. Guide Through the Stages of Recovery from Emotionally Abusive Relationships with a Narcissist

Benedict Daniel

Table of Contents

Introduction

Many people enter into a relationship with high hopes, expectations, and happiness. The thought of sharing your life, your goals, and your dreams with another person is exciting. Even though you know the journey will not be smooth, there will be ups and downs, but you are confident you will pull through and surmount everything life throws at you.

This is the expectation of everyone at the beginning of a new relationship. It is, however, not so if you are with a narcissistic partner. They charm you with sweet talk and charisma, and they are confident—which many people (women, especially) find attractive. Hence, before you know it, you are entangled in a romantic relationship with them.

In time, however, you start seeing your partner for who they are. You've showered them with so much love, but you receive nothing in return. You've invested yourself heavily into the relationship with the hope that your partner will take the clue and work harder, as well. They hurt you, lash out at you, make a mountain out of a molehill, and never seem interested even though they say it with their mouths. You have confronted them several times. They either promise to change or twist your brain around and turn everything on you. They tell you that you are suffocating them, that you are not giving them breathing space in the relationship. And so, you start second-guessing yourself, not sure if you can believe yourself or not. They never accept they are wrong and will manipulate every situation and opportunity for discussion such that everything comes back on you.

If the above sounds like what you are experiencing, I am pretty sure you know you are in a relationship with a narcissist. Yes, you read right. This is the aim of putting together this life-changing manual. Does the following describe you?

- You are emotionally, even physically detached from your immediate environment.

- You find yourself walking on eggshells around people. It could be your narcissist partner, your friends, or your family. This is an indirect result of the abuse on you.

- You sacrifice a lot, like your needs (physical and emotional) and even sometimes your safety to satisfy your abusive partner.

- Your stress level has increased significantly.

- You struggle with health issues like weight loss or gain, difficulty sleeping, terrifying nightmares, etc. that did not exist before the relationship.

- You suddenly start trying to please everyone.

- To trust others now becomes an issue and you are always anxious about other people's intentions.

- You tend to be alone, isolated from friends and loved ones. This is not surprising, as many abusers tend to keep their victims away from those who care about them.

If the above describes you, you are a victim of narcissistic relationship abuse. The good news is that you can get help. That is the sole aim of putting together this book. Before you lose yourself and your personality entirely to your abusive partner, you can take helpful steps. These are steps that will allow you to get a hold of your life, recover, and move past the trauma of the abusive relationship.

This is a detailed manual that will hold you by the hand

in helping you recover from a narcissistic relationship. We will explain all the tactics of the narcissist, so you can protect yourself against their whims. In addition, we will walk you through the breakup, while preparing yourself for the aftermath of fallout and anything the narcissist might have planned for you.

Finally, there will be practical steps to help you through the recovery period. Leaving a narcissistic relationship is not as simple as leaving a normal relationship (even though all breakups are tough). However, due to the psychological damage and trauma that the abusive partner has caused, you need all the help you can get. Besides, when you leave a narcissist, you are usually drained, and you feel a lot less than yourself. This makes it important to consciously subscribe to any assistance you can find in restoring your sanity. This is what we will offer you.

Part of our aim in writing this book is to make your recovery process smooth. We hope that you can achieve this by the time you take the bold step to break up with a narcissist.

There is hope, and you can be free!

Chapter 1: Basics of Narcissistic Abuse

There are many people in relationships with narcissists, yet it does not dawn on them the damaging effect of their partner's behavior until it has already taken its toll. This is not surprising, as a narcissist's abuse can alter the victim's perception of reality.

Being with a narcissist is hard because of their exaggerated sense of self-importance, which hurts the relationship and the other people in their life. To a narcissist, the people around them are the fuel they need to boost their ego. The sad part is that many victims of narcissism might not be able to detect these problems. This is due to the charming nature of the narcissist, and the tricks with which they can deceive people into accepting them.

In any area of life, dealing with a narcissist—maybe in a relationship or as a family member—can be tedious, frustrating, and exhausting. When you are in a relationship with a narcissist who has become abusive, it can be especially devastating. This is because such abuse is sneaky, can be damaging both physically and emotionally, and worst of all, might not be easy to recognize.

Most of these relationships likely started well—I bet you would not choose to be in a relationship with an abuser in the first place. People with these tendencies start off as loving and charming, as long as they want something from you. Bear in mind that the people with narcissistic tendencies do not become abusive overnight.

With time, however, you can easily pick out a narcissist. This is because they become skillful at enslaving people's minds and will with their language. In a bid to prevent you from realizing their effect on you, narcissists have a way of manipulating their victim's emotions. With this, they can easily make their victim take responsibility for everything that goes wrong in the relationship.

The narcissistic abuse, however, is a form of thought manipulation in which the narcissist employs the use of language to manipulate someone. The aim of this is to take control of the person's mind and will such that the narcissist can use it for his selfish desires. In fact, the aim of the narcissist is to get the victim to do any of the following:

- Question their decision-making ability

- Lose faith in their own judgment

- Capitalize on their faults and errors

- Doubt their friends and families and others that support them

- Prioritize making the narcissist happy and giving the narcissist what he wants

The Narcissist Abuse Syndrome

More often than not, victims of narcissistic abuse see

themselves as the problem. This is because of the success of the narcissist in manipulating their will and emotions. As a result, victims often will be obsessed with their inadequacies, shortcomings, failures, etc. The victim tries desperately to look for a solution to these issues since, according to the narcissist, it is the cause of his misery. The victim accepts responsibility for all shortcomings, and every innocent thing they do is questioned.

The victim often ends up confused in the midst of this occurrence. She is so obsessed with looking for an explanation and solution for why her partner treats her so bad—why they cannot seem to communicate well, and he is always miserable or angry and finds fault with everything she does, etc. She accepts all this since the narcissist successfully used tactics like gaslighting and rage to manipulate her.

The continuous interaction with the narcissist has made them idolize him. In other words, he is faultless, while they are the cause of everything going wrong. This fills the victim with self-condemnation and, when asked, she makes statements like:

- We only quarrel once a while, we get along most of

- the time.

- It is all my fault.

- How can I stop making him so mad?

- Will he still love me despite this?

- Why am I so damaged that I have to keep upsetting him?

- It is all my fault that he gets so mad.

We have established that the narcissist does succeed in manipulating the will and mind of their victim. This explains why a careful examination of the narcissist's thinking pattern shows a biased sense of responsibility. For instance, the victim falsely assumes that:

- She does not know how to make her partner secure.

- She is clueless about getting herself to stop upsetting him.

- All the bad and horrible things he has done like yelling, name-calling, etc., is her fault

- She pushes him to the wall, so if he doesn't get over minor things, it is justified.

- She forced him out to other women with her behavior.

Many at times, what the victim thinks and feels about herself, the problem, and the narcissist, is to a great extent a reflection of how the narcissist thinks and feels. In other words, he has succeeded in manipulating her to think and believe what he wants. This is why the term "emotional manipulation" and narcissistic abuse go hand in hand.

The Nature and Effect of Narcissistic Abuse

If you were once a victim of narcissistic abuse, you need to understand the nature, effect, and concept of narcissistic abuse syndrome. This is vital for your complete healing and restoring of your sanity. Bear in mind that a person with a narcissistic personality disorder, (NPD) will not feel guilty for using and hurting the victim.

A narcissist takes pleasure in hurting, inflicting pain, and manipulating others for their gain, without an iota of guilt or remorse. To a narcissist, only weak and inferior persons feel remorseful. On the other side, however, a narcissist is weak. And to him, mutual caring and human love are deceptive illusions. As a result, he develops a false sense of importance in which he sees himself as superhuman.

Despite the self-serving nature of the narcissist, they need other people to validate this impulse. In other words, they need the input of others to boost their ego and buttress the fact that they are super humans, way above everyone else. Even though narcissistic abuse expresses itself in most forms of human relationships, it is most common in a romantic relationship. This is because love generally makes us vulnerable, which makes people easier to manipulate.

A narcissist's abuse can come in any form—mental, physical, emotional, mental, etc.—all with the same aim: control, and self-validation. Narcissists, in a bid to prove that they are superior to others, will resort to abusive behaviors. With this, he will manipulate others, especially his partner, to do things that serve him.

Often, the abuse on the part of the narcissist is calculated and deliberate. This way, the victim questions their worth and accepts responsibility. This is why narcissistic abuse is so dangerous, especially when the brainwashing has gotten to the point where the victim accepts that she only exists to take care of his victim and his ego. If this goes on for long, it could lead to a complete loss of sense of self and worth.

Psychological and Emotional Harm of Narcissistic Abuse

When in a relationship with a narcissist for too long, it is possible for the victim to start accepting and believing the distorted reality their partner has set. This is not surprising, as the narcissist is fond of using manipulation, rage or outburst, gaslighting, lying, and derive joy from overstepping the boundaries to mess with the victim's sense of reasoning. This, in turn, makes the victim falsely believe their partner truly cares for them. In reality, however, it is near impossible for a narcissist to feel real love. This is because of the lack of empathy and a deep need for admiration.

As a result, partners of narcissists can experience traumatic and emotional harm. This might come as a result of the verbal and emotional abuse, the coercions, etc., which all work to deplete their self-esteem. Being with a narcissist can so significantly traumatize a person that the victim can develop symptoms of anxiety and depression or post-traumatic stress disorder.

This is why many of the symptoms of post-traumatic stress disorder (PTSD) is common with narcissist abuse syndrome. Some of these are:

- Unhealthy thoughts about themselves and the world around them

- Flashbacks and nightmares

- A feeling of detachment from others

- Staying away from people or situations that trigger the trauma

- Poor concentration and sleep pattern

- Visible reactions to whatever triggers trauma

How Does the Narcissist Manipulate the Victim?

As established above, the narcissist has several weapons in their arsenal to manipulate their victim. We thought it important to explain the basics of some of their tactics such as the narcissist rage (or outburst), gaslighting, their love for violating boundaries, and the concept of reciprocation. The knowledge of these weapons will help you guard yourself against every whim of the narcissist.

Understanding Narcissist Rage

Have you ever seen a two-year-old throw a tantrum? It appears from nowhere, as if triggered by some unseen forces. It creates a scene, without regard to the people around. This in turn leaves others in a state of shock.

One of the priorities of a narcissist is gaining admiration, love, and affection from others. People with narcissistic personality disorder will use everything within their capacity to try and achieve this. At times, however, when they fail to receive the love and admiration they desire, they resort to what is called the narcissist outburst. What are the symptoms of a narcissist outburst?

It could be gentle and nonviolent, such as:

- Vocal disagreement

- Visible irritation

- Withdrawal or silent treatment to punish the offender

- Head shaking, etc.,

Severe and violent symptoms include:

- An outburst of physical violence

- Vocal outrage

It should be pointed out that there is a clear-cut difference between regular anger and a display of rage by a narcissist. Many at times, the rage and outburst of a narcissist is baseless and triggered by an occurrence that would not provoke such reaction in others. This is why narcissists are often seen as selfish losers. Anger, on the other hand, is often triggered by a rational cause and should subside when expressed.

Heinz Kohut came up with the term "narcissist rage" in the year 1972 in his book *The Analysis of the Self*. The rage of the narcissist is usually triggered when he feels he is being attacked by another person. Vanity, grandiose self-worth, entitlement, etc., are common with a narcissist. When any of these is challenged, it leads to a perceived form of injury called "Narcissistic Injury," a threat to their importance and self-worth.

For the narcissist to survive, they need to be constantly admired, complimented, and adored. They are clouded with the illusion that people should worship them. As a result, they are known to form a parasitic type of relationship with others in which they feed on them to keep their self-esteem up.

As a result, any challenge or disagreement from another party is considered a threat, criticism, attack, and rejection. This is why they react fiercely to such attack and lash out at the source of their provocation.

Causes of Narcissistic Outburst

When their Confidence is Questioned

Many times, people with narcissistic tendencies will place irrational demand and expectations on their partner or kids. At times when they are challenged, they consider it as an attack on their ego. This is because they cannot accept the fact that they are wrong, imperfect, or have shortcomings. This makes them resort to outbursts in a bid to regain their sense of superiority.

Insult to Their Self-esteem

When someone reveals the weakness or imperfection of a narcissist, the narcissist is engulfed with an overwhelming sense of shame. This triggers an outburst of anger toward the person who revealed the weakness. This rage or outburst is often an attempt to exert revenge. And unlike anger, the outburst does not die down until the narcissist feels the threat has been dealt with.

Altered Sense of Self

This explains the fake sense of identity and capacity of the narcissist. There are times when the narcissist feels undeserving of love from the people around him. This might spring up from childhood experiences. As a result, the narcissist resorts to the superficial relationship in an effort to nurture his idealized sense of importance. Should anything, however, make the partner doubt the authenticity and dedication of the narcissist, he resorts to outburst as a means of self-defense.

Understanding the Gaslighting Technique

One of the most brutal weapons in the arsenal of a narcissist is gaslighting. The narcissist uses gaslighting to confuse and distort the victim's perception of reality. As a result, victims question their sanity and the authenticity of their memory. In other words, gaslighting makes you wonder if you can trust yourself.

With gaslighting, the victim turns to the abuser for what they thought to be real, and with time, he is considered as the authority in their life. Gaslighting is so subtle that it is hard to recognize. With most emotional abuse, a careful and rational analysis of the situation can help unveil it. In other forms of emotional abuse, the abuser shames you, criticizes your effort, stops all form of communication, keeps you from the people you love, gives you the cold-shoulder treatment, etc.

Gaslighting is, however, not this obvious. The narcissist will not resort to obvious abuse technique. However, he will manipulate, twist, and misinterpret the facts in order to get you confused. He might succeed as he has tricked you into doubting your sanity. Controlling another person is not easy, which makes gaslighting a tricky form of abuse.

There are many people who are a victim of gaslighting. To free yourself from this sneaky form of abuse, it is important to understand how to recognize it. But before that, why do narcissists use gaslighting?

- Gaslighting gives them control over their victim.

- With gaslighting, they can manipulate you into believing that they are right, that your perception of reality is faulty.

- Gaslighting helps them make you lose trust in your feelings and sense of reality.

- They use gaslighting as a tool to reduce the gravity of any situation.

- Gaslighting helps them play the victim and avoid responsibility and scolding.

- They use gaslighting as a tool to shy away from fulfilling a promise once made.

- With gaslighting, they can cook up stories, events, and conversations that never took place.

To also help you understand the game plan of the

narcissist when they employ gaslighting, it is important to understand how they talk.

- You will hear narcissist say things like, "This did not happen, that was not what I said. It is not that bad; remember, you said..."

- They will say you are paranoid when you seek to understand things.

- They will say you are blowing things out of proportion.

- They will tell you what someone else said about you that is not true, all in a bid to make you feel the person does not like you.

- They will make something up to water down your confidence so to prevent you from speaking up.

Watch out for the toxic and convert ones, as they play on the fact that you love them and use it to manipulate you. They are really tricky because, on the surface, they are so harmless. Watch out for speech like, "It is not like that, my love. I am only worried about you, which is why I am..."

- They will tell you that you are hallucinating.

- They will tell you that you have a problem with something. For instance, if the abuser is constantly fond of flirting with the opposite sex and you have been upset about it several times, the gaslighter will say something like, "You seem to have problem with trust."

- Looking at the phrases above, it sounds completely normal with nothing out of the ordinary. Yet, as innocent as it seems, it can alter one's sense of reality.

Unveiling the Gaslighter Personality

Considering how diabolical gaslighting is, why would anyone think it is acceptable to do to someone else? This practice is specific to people who try to control others using any means. It is common among people who do not believe in being wrong and will do anything to prove that others are wrong, instead. Narcissism and gaslighting go hand in hand because the abuser makes everything about their needs, and brainwashes the victim to think that they are helping them. Yet, a careful analysis of the relationship reveals that their action is building the narcissist's ego.

Boundary Process

Boundaries are a big turn-off to the narcissist. Setting boundaries is like dealing a big blow to a narcissist, as they take this as rejection. If you object and say no to their request, they take it as a rejection of their needs and feelings. They take it as a personal rejection, which does not go down well with them. Have in mind that the narcissist always feels they have the right to whatever they desire. Hence, rejection to a narcissist means that you do not care about them.

It is just like a kid who wants to play with her friends outside. Mummy objects, and says she must do the dishes before going out. The child throws a tantrum and concludes that mummy is mean. This is the same way a narcissist takes rejection. Their emotional state is not mature, which affects how they relate to the world. In the same manner, rejecting their advances means you do not want them to feel better. They do not bother to reason that what they are after might be uncomfortable to others, or just plain hurtful. All that occupies their mind is what they are after. This is why the narcissist does not do well with boundaries.

Narcissists are usually controlled by their emotions and fulfillment. In other words, they are after what they can get, as well as how something makes them feel. When there is a strong boundary, however, they feel rejected since the avenue of getting what they want is blocked. A person with a strong boundary already has a strong wall of defense, which will prevent them from getting to the person. In other words, there is no room for manipulation, abuse, etc. This is why the relationship with the narcissist is pointless.

It is important to point out that narcissists are not attracted to empaths alone. Narcissists are also drawn to people with class, social influence, people with money, and other desirable qualities. Narcissists will play their tricks on everyone, even though they will not work on everyone. The most vulnerable people are those with poor boundaries. These are people without a clear definition of what they will not accept. People with a strong limit, on the other hand, draw the line immediately. Once a narcissist pushes the boundary, the line is drawn.

A narcissist will surely push the boundaries, as it is in their DNA. A narcissist has a distorted view of the world.

Boundaries have no meaning to them, as they believe their feeling is everyone's feeling. And a narcissist's feeling is basically negative and self-centered. Besides, there will come a time in the relationship or interaction where a narcissist will accuse you of causing their feelings through whatever you said or did. This will be followed by the narcissist's rage, outbursts, pointless accusations, and inevitable abuse. A person with poor boundaries might be tricked into trying to figure out what his fault was and how to make amends. A person with a strong boundary, on the other hand, will severe the tie. An individual who does not give the narcissist excuses does not interest them.

I bet you now understand why boundaries turn narcissists off. If you let them slide just once, they will always come back at you with a strong force. This, to them, is a weakness, an opportunity to exploit you— which they will do until they get what they want. Have you ever seen a dog desperate to get out of a crate? All they need is a single weakness and failure in the structure. They will push and stretch this weakness until it gives way for them to escape. The weakness does not have to be substantial. This is why you cannot let your guard down once you suspect you are with a narcissist.

Reciprocation

One of the worst mistakes you can make in life is telling a narcissist you love him. This is because you just handed him the weapon he needs to punish and make your life miserable. Besides, a narcissist is full of hatred for himself, which he will transfer to all those who make the mistake of loving them.

This is usually difficult for people with a compassionate nature. This is because the more nice, generous, and compassionate you are to a narcissist, the more you will be punished. Normally, when you love someone, you expect to be loved back. This only holds true for sane people—not the narcissist. As a result, the nicer and sweeter you are to a narcissist, the more hurt, pain, disappointment, and misery you can expect in return.

None of your needs will be acknowledged, let alone met. Expect no appreciation or reward for your effort. Even if he compliments you, it is not genuine. To a narcissist, you are just a tool, a pawn, a means to an end. This is why he will never reciprocate any good thing you do. As a result, bending over backwards to satisfy the narcissist will only end up compounding your hurt.

A narcissist, however, will be on their best behavior when they have boundaries. Hence, people with healthy boundaries and limits that are enforced know how to put a narcissist in their place.

Chapter 2: How to Survive a Narcissist Relationship

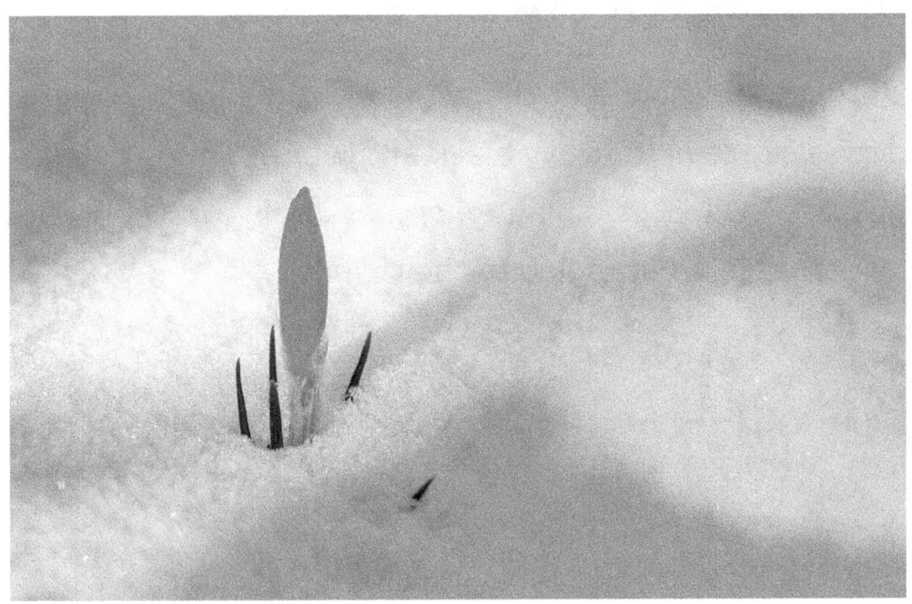

Getting entangled with a narcissist is easy because they are skilled at hiding who they are. They are people with attractive traits like confidence and other charming characteristics. This makes it easy to be lured into dating a narcissist.

In desperation to hold tight to the relationship, you might justify their actions by saying they had a bad day, and the next day will not be like that. You might even discuss it with them, and they wave it aside, making you feel it is nothing or that you think too much. You, however, will begin to realize that it does not get better and the relationship is draining you.

You need to know that the signs of a relationship with a narcissist are not always black and white. This is because they are skilled at hiding who they really are until they have you fully entangled in their web.

Signs You are in a Relationship with a Narcissist

Note that narcissists are skillful at hiding their true colors. As a result, you need to be aware of how the mind of a narcissist works for you to identify one. In fact, people with narcissistic personality can be recognized because of the following characteristics, as all they do will revolve around this.

- *Entitlement*: They believe in getting what they want.

- *One-mindedness*: To a narcissist, only a single point of view exists—theirs.

- *Absence of empathy*: They cannot understand how others feel due to their low emotional quotient.

- *No sense of proportion:* All you need to set a narcissist off is a slight mistake, and you see them making a mountain out of a molehill.

There are many signs that will reveal you are in a relationship with a narcissist. The four characteristics discussed above are usually the underlying cause. Here are the signs you will see when dating one:

They Often Threaten You

Watch out for threats from your partner. It might be a threat to leave you, to blackmail you, etc. It is usually common with a narcissist. Watch out for statements like:

- "If you do not do this by _____, consider this relationship over."

- "Everyone will know what kind of person you are."

- "I am better off without you, go ahead and leave."

Excessive Need for Attention and Validation

If your partner has a high need for validation, there is a tendency you are dealing with a narcissist. They will try every means to get your attention. To a narcissist, external validation is important for them to feel good and wanted.

The sad part, however, is that it does not count much. Even though they so crave validation and approval from you, it is never enough. No matter how much you let them know you care for them and approve of them, it doesn't soothe them. This is due to the fact that they do not see anyone truly loving them. This can be traced to the root of a narcissist because despite being self-absorbed, they are insecure deep-down—hence the desire for more and more approval.

A Huge Need for Control

A narcissist is never contented with life. This makes him try all in his capacity to mold things to his liking. As a result of this, they have a compulsion for control. Their sense of entitlement also makes it logical for them to want to be in control.

A narcissist has an idealized way in which people should act. When people fail to behave as expected, it upsets them. Since you've already deviated, they are clueless about what to expect next, which throws them off-balance.

The narcissist wants you to act and do as they please so they can reach their idealized conclusion. To them, you are just a pawn to achieve their selfish desire—a robot that should be controlled and told what to do!

Inability to Accept Responsibility

While narcissists strive to be in control, they also have the tendency to dodge responsibility for the outcome. This only changes if the result goes as expected; otherwise, they feel inadequate and place all the blame on you. Accepting fault is never in their nature as they just have to deflect.

There are times the blame could be generalized—the government, the law enforcement agent, the caregivers, etc. Other times, a particular person could be the object of his blame, like his parents, his colleague, his boss, etc. Most times, however, the blame falls on the person most emotionally close to the narcissist.

They cannot do without blaming, as it helps keep up with their idealized sense of perfection.

Perfectionism

In the narcissist's world, they are perfect. As a result, they expect you and everyone else to be perfect. Narcissists have this invisible script well planned out in their head, dictating how things should go. Events, life, and people around them must follow this carefully crafted script, just like they want it.

This, without a doubt, is an impossible demand, which eventually makes the narcissist miserable and dissatisfied.

Emotional Reasoning

You might be frustrated about the behavior of your partner. You tried everything in your effort to explain to him and make him see how much pain and suffering he is causing you. You expect him will adjust if he understands how much he hurts you. But since a narcissist is only caught up in his world, your explanations make little to no sense to him. Even if he admits he understands, he really does not.

Thus to a narcissist, their actions and decisions are usually based on how they feel. The only reason they need to get the latest Lamborghini is how driving it makes them feel. They are not bothered by the fact that it is a burden on the family and budget. At the slightest provocation and discomfort, a narcissist could quit his job with the hope of moving to another one or starting a business. To a narcissist, their problem can only be solved by something or someone else, not themselves.

Fear and Anxiety

The life of a narcissist revolves around fear, yet for most of them, this fear is deeply buried. They fear being wrong, being seen as incapable, not being accepted, etc. They fear being fired, being tested, being considered inadequate. It is because of this fear that a narcissist hardly trusts anyone.

The deeper your relationship gets, the more he becomes suspicious of you. Narcissists have a phobia for true intimacy as it makes them vulnerable, which could expose their weak points. All your assurance and reassurance makes no difference, as their imperfection is a personal turnoff.

An Inability to be Vulnerable

Since a narcissist cannot truly process feelings, and since they always need to protect their image, it is difficult for them to truly connect with others. Since they are full of themselves and their ways, they cannot consider things from another person's perspective. Emotionally, they are lonely, which makes them needy.

When a relationship does not give them what they want, they pull the plug as soon as possible and jump to the next one. Wired deep in their DNA is the need to always make everything as they want it, have someone feel their pain and sympathize with them. On the contrary, however, they are not capable of responding to someone else's need.

The Narcissist and the Empath

That ancient law of physics tells us that opposite poles attract. This does not apply to the world of physics alone, but humans as well. Unfortunately, however, the attraction between a narcissist and an empath is a dangerous and painful one. This is because their relationship is the definition of all kinds of abuse, exploitation, violation, and neglect. The painful part is that only one partner suffers it.

Empaths are known to be kind, generous, and loving

people, with the capacity to relate with other people's emotions. You do not have to be an empath to be unlucky to be in a relationship with a narcissist. However, the rate at which empaths get entangled with narcissists is pretty high, which makes this particular dynamic deserve some investigation.

Who are the Empaths?

Empaths find it pretty easy to relate to other people's feelings. It can be said that they truly feel what others feel because of their unique ability to tune in to the emotions of others. They are sensitive and caring, and will care for others at the expense of taking care of themselves. This is why they attract narcissists.

What About the Narcissists?

On the other hand, narcissists are selfish, emotionless people who have trouble relating to the feelings of others. They do not even recognize that others have feelings, let alone bother to consider those feelings. A narcissist, in short, lacks the true ability to empathize with others.

To think that these two completely different people will be attracted to each other is a lot to take in. Surprisingly, however, these two form a solid, unbreakable yet toxic bond.

How do Empaths and Narcissist Attract Each Other?

A careful examination of the kind of personality that narcissists and empaths have reveal why they are attracted to each other. Empaths are the definition of what is lacking in the narcissists: supportive, emotional, caring, and hospitable. The narcissist wants what he does not have and seeks to get these things from those who have them. The empath, being selfless, willingly opens herself to the narcissist like the way a bright flower attracts a butterfly. This, to the narcissist, is a source of emotion he can leech off for as long as he wants. The empath, true to her nature, is willing to give and give as needed.

This is the kind of relationship that exists between these two extreme personalities.

One might wonder, why on earth is the gentle, loving empath attracted to the coldhearted and selfish narcissist? This is because, at the onset, the narcissist gives off a vibe so strong that it is difficult, if not impossible, for the empath to ignore. The way a magnet will spot, attract, and cling to the tiniest piece of iron in a piece of rubble, the empath is drawn to the narcissist.

Empaths, being emotionally-sensitive personalities, are attracted to the strong emotions that narcissists give. He might, however, appear to be difficult to read, despite his strong and intense vibe. The empath is drawn to this in spite of the difficulty they may have figuring him out. In an attempt to get to know him and everything about him, the narcissist reveals a tale of his ordeal and abuse (real or fake). He also proceeds to blow his own horn, making himself seem so wonderful, irresistible to resist. This ends up snaring the unguarded empath, making her fall for his tactics.

One might want to argue that empaths should know better than to fall for the deceptiveness of the narcissist. This is true, as empaths are known to be in tune with the emotions of others. Hence, the empaths can actually sense that something does not add up about this fellow, which often happens during the first interaction. However, the empath is drawn to how broken and wounded he is, and the empath fails to listen to all warning signals and falls for him. It should be noted that the narcissist is truly broken and wounded inside. Hence this is neither an act on the narcissist's part (even though there might be lies or exaggerations) nor a mistake on the part of the empath. Narcissists are skilled at appearing helpless and lost, which is true as they really are.

The fatal mistake of the empath, however, is thinking she can fix him. The narcissist cannot be helped.

One might ask why such a deadly combination?

The narcissist will make the empath believe that besides her, no other person can help him. At other times, he might even make her believe that she's doing a terrific job of caring for him. This makes the empath happy, as she feels she is fulfilling her basic need: to truly help others. She falls for this, as the narcissist is skilled at pressing someone's emotional buttons and cajoling them to get what they want. It is a doomed codependent relationship that is centered on fulfilling the superficial needs of only one party—a party that can never truly be satisfied. To understand this better, imagine what a futile effort it is if you fetch water with a basket.

It is also important to point out that, in a way, the relationship also fulfills the empath's need—although it doesn't seem to be the case, as the empath is more prone to abuse and hurt in the relationship. However, she has consciously set herself for the hurt since she prides herself in deriving fulfillment from helping someone who does not care about getting better. It is when an empath recognizes this that she can break free from the entanglement she is in. The empath needs to know that the narcissist only seems to have power over her because she makes it so. She can walk out or choose to continue in the relationship.

There are many narcissists out there who are achievers, but they have their disorder as a challenge to be surmounted. The empath is drawn to this and sees it as an opportunity to bring out her nurturing attribute. No matter how much she tries to ignore him, her desire to nurture can make it feel like an obligation. He is lost without her. Abandoning him will be cruel and inhumane of her, since his state is not his fault. And truly, we admit that a narcissist cannot help how their brain is wired. He might have been abused as a kid. He might have experienced rejection from a tender age. None of this was likely the narcissist's fault. The empath also needs to understand that the state and condition of the narcissist is not her fault, either. Hence, she does not have to be punished for the mistake of another person as well, except she deliberately chose to be in a codependent relationship.

This is why most empaths miss it, the lack of willpower to let go of people they feel need their help. Her sense of logic is faulty—thinking that if she does not help him, no one will.

Knowing When it's Time to Leave a Narcissist

What a toxic relationship, being with a narcissist! You might be fed up of complaining about their shortcomings and what they did to upset you.

Since, eventually, you will end up apologizing.

You are fascinated by a life in which you are free from them, in which you are with someone that values and respect you. Yet, you cannot seem to summon the courage to leave them, and you still love them.

The good news, however, is that another life *is* possible.

No matter how deep a relationship you are in with the narcissist, even if you share children, you can get your life back. You are neither bound to be a caregiver to the narcissist, neither do you have to put up with the abuse.

It is all about understanding how to leave them. You just need the courage and strength to rise above the manipulations and crafty ways in which they hold you. Even if the thought of leaving them seems scary, you can get away.

Understand How and When to Leave a Narcissist

To understand the right time, as well as how to leave a narcissist, it is important to explore how the abuse distorted your sense of being. Over time, in the relationship, the narcissist completely shut off your dreams. You had no voice, which made you question your life and existence in general.

This, however, is part of the narcissist's game to make you get lost in their identity. It is a one-sided relationship that makes you lose yourself into them. As a result, you find yourself obsessed with them and nothing else, rather than seeking ways to improve your own life, family, and career.

If this sounds familiar, then you have lost your sense of sense and identity to the narcissist. This is a huge sign you need to leave your partner. Besides that, here are other red flags that show you need to get out of your relationship with a narcissist as soon as possible:

Your mental health is suffering: All the constant longing to please them, your efforts to make the relationship work, etc. is making you anxious and depressed. You could also have other health deterioration.

You are losing your self-worth: This is common with victims of narcissistic abuse. Spending too much time in a relationship with a narcissist makes the victim stop caring and valuing themselves.

A consistent cycle of fault: A common characteristic of the narcissist is repeating mistakes, apologizing, and promising it will never happen again yet repeating the cycle. It might be cheating, calling you names, etc. Bear in mind that the probability of change is low.

The relationship is focused on the narcissist: It is what they do. They love the attention and admiration they get from blowing their own horn. Besides, he will hardly care about your opinions. Even though he allows you to share it, he is not genuinely interested.

You do the hard work in the relationship: *Remember* that a narcissist is mainly after what he can get from you and the relationship. As a result, there will not be any major input in the relationship, except when it favors him. If you are having a difficult time, do not expect a narcissist to be there for you. It is not how they are wired!

Even though the writing on the wall is clear, the decision to leave the relationship is entirely up to you. But keep in mind that the narcissist will make you feel that you are lost without them. However, summoning the courage to leave can be the turning point in your life.

The Concept of Gaslighting

Gaslighting is an abuse that is common in a narcissistic relationship. Having laid the foundation in the first chapter, this section will shed light on tactics used in gaslighting.

We established that the narcissist makes you second-guess yourself, your perception of reality, and memory. They make you wonder if you are even sane, since you are left confused and dazed. This section will explore the tactics the narcissist uses in gaslighting victims.

Hence, if you want to know if you are being gaslighted, watch out for one or more of the following:

Constantly Lies to You

Narcissists who employ gaslighting as a weapon are habitual liars. Even when you are convinced of their lie, they will refuse to back down. This is because lying is the cornerstone of their behavior, which can appear so real and convincing. They are so skilled at lying that you begin to second-guess yourself.

They Discredit You to Others

This involves spreading rumors about your behavior to discredit you in the eyes of others. You accuse them of unfaithfulness while they go ahead and tell everyone you are paranoid and overly jealous. The sad part is, many people innocently side with the abuser without knowing the full story.

On the other hand, the gaslighter feeds with you with

wrong and false information. He will do all in his power to make you believe this, to achieve what he wants.

Deflects the Subject of Conversation

When you question him about his whereabouts the previous night, he asks you why that is important. This is an effort to change the topic, rather than addressing the issue. If you are persistent, they will surely lie to cover up their tracks.

Discredit Your Thoughts and Feelings

They tell you that you are blowing things out of proportion, that you are overreacting, that you are too sensitive. This is all an effort to discredit and trivialize your feelings and concerns. They successfully end up making you think you are wrong. When you spend more time with someone who does not acknowledge your thoughts and feelings, you also end up losing faith in yourself.

Use Compassionate Words to Manipulate You

Have you ever heard these words?

"You mean too much to me for me to intentionally hurt you."

They sound sincere and genuine. However, a gaslighter will resort to this technique when you call them out in a bid to smooth the situation over. They know you want to hear nice words, so they will use them. These words, however, are not genuine, especially when the narcissist just repeats the same mistake.

Examples of Gaslighting in Relationships

Countering: Here, the abuser distorts what happens and makes the victim question the situation with statements like:

- "You are getting old and losing your memory."

- "That is not what happened."

- "Are you sure you remembered correctly?"

Withholding: Here, the narcissist tactically dismisses your point/argument. They might pretend they do not understand. Watch out for things like:

- "You are imagining things."

- "You are not making sense."

Repetitive Question: With repetitive questions, the

abuser makes the victim doubt what they know, think, or feel. He asks you:

- "Is that so?"

- "Are you sure?"

Trivializing: The abuser makes a remark to belittle the victim's feelings. You hear things like:

- "You are so sensitive."

- "You are blowing things out of proportion."

Revealing Hidden Thoughts of Others: This is where the abuser makes up something (which could be true or false) that others are saying or thinking about the victim. The aim is to hurt the victim, or make them doubt themselves. Consider this example:

"Even though you meant well by coming to the party, I saw Jane and Natasha rolling their eyes when you came in."

Dealing With Emotional Abuse from a Narcissist

When we are hurt, frustrated, or angry, we might be

guilty of abuse like judging, controlling, criticizing, etc. Emotional abuse from a narcissist is, however, on a different level. There are emotional abuses from a narcissist that you cannot spot easily, like gaslighting. They could threaten and intimidate you for them to have control over you.

Narcissistic abuse can look innocent (for example, silence) and can be extreme (for example, violence). Additionally, rarely will you see a narcissist take responsibility for their actions. They have a way of denying facts and passing the blame to the victim. They also lack the capacity to feel guilty.

In dealing with emotional abuse from a narcissist, it is important to understand the intent of their abuse, which is power. Bear in mind that the narcissist wants to control and dominate you. Besides that, they need you to feel guilty and ashamed. The abuse creates a sense of superiority in them, a tactic to hide their real feelings of inferiority. This simple knowledge can be your ticket to breaking free from emotional abuse. Ever seen a bully? They are arrogant, with an inflated sense of worth. Their worst nightmare is being seen as weak and humiliated. This knowledge will go a long way in preventing the abuse of a narcissist from getting to you.

Errors in Dealing with Emotional Abuse

If you do not know the tactics and intent of a narcissist, you will naturally react in some ways that are not healthy. Be sure to watch out for the following:

Pleading: This gives the impression that you are weak. When you plead, you give the narcissist the license to treat you with disrespect.

Withdrawal: While withdrawal might make you feel good temporarily, it will not deal with the abuse effectively.

Complaining and Criticizing: In a bid not to appear weak and insecure, they put forward a tough skin. They lash at you, criticize you as if they are strong, yet they cannot take it in return. Hence, resorting to these tactics could provoke anger.

Self-Blame: Accepting responsibility for the abuser's action by trying to be perfect and working on yourself is futile. Bear in mind that you are only responsible for your behavior, and not that of others. Part of the root cause of a narcissist's vindictive behavior to you is insecurity, not you.

Denial: Assuming that the abuse will stop or go away with time is a terrible mistake. And no, they are not having a bad day! Stop making excuses for them. Rationalizing abuse is like condoning it, giving it a fertile ground to germinate. The more you condone it, the longer it goes on, which makes you weaker.

Now that we have set a foundation on how not to react to a narcissist's abuse, the next section discusses how to deal with emotional abuse from a narcissist.

Confront the Abuse

This is not about fighting or arguing; it will not work. Rather, we mean speaking up for yourself and expressing yourself clearly and effectively. The more you put up with abuse, the more your self-esteem pays for it.

Be Clear on Your Rights

Even if you do not know, I am telling you today that you have specific rights. You have rights to your feelings and choices, a right to decline to go anywhere you don't want to go, a right not to be yelled at, a right not to be taken for granted, a right to say no without feeling guilty, etc.

Putting up with long-term abuse can make your self-esteem diminish so much that you easily give up your rights.

Be Assertive

This is not about being aggressive; it involves knowing how to express yourself without fear of any consequence. In other words, you should be comfortable speaking your mind. If you do not have an answer for a request, tell him. Let him know you don't like being criticized and tell him to stop. Do not be intimidated into accepting what they tell you—reveal your stance.

Have Clear Boundaries

Boundaries are like personal constitution with which you should be treated. Bear in mind that you deserve what you allow. This calls for clearly knowing your boundaries and expressing them to the narcissist. Communicate your boundaries in black and white, as people cannot read your mind. If you do not want to be visited after 8 pm, make it known. Let him know you will not be yelled at or blackmailed.

Set Consequences

We established in the first chapter that narcissists hate boundaries. As a result, do not expect it to go over well with him. This is why you need consequences, should your boundaries be neglected. Be sure not to have empty threats, but a specific measure to protect yourself. For instance, requesting for a restraining order should any of your boundaries be violated!

The narcissist tends to see themselves as smart, but you can outsmart them. These measures can go a long way in protecting you and keeping your sanity intact from the emotional abuse of a narcissist.

Chapter 3: How to Defeat a Narcissist

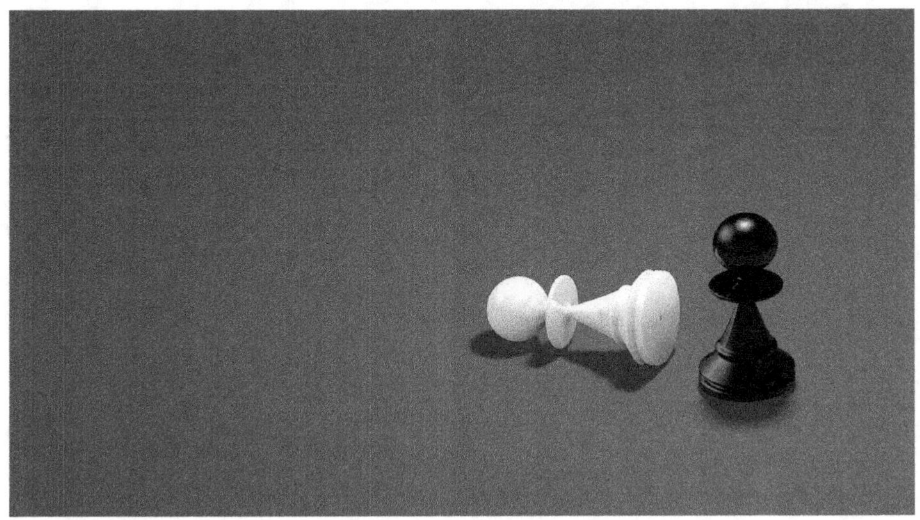

Remember that a narcissist is calculated in their actions and behaviors. As a result, you need to be strategic if you want to get your life back. This chapter will explore a proven strategy that will help you break free from the shackles the narcissist has on you. But before proceeding to that, it is important to understand the mind of a narcissist.

How to Understand the Playing Field That Narcissists Thrive On

It is hard, if not impossible, for people in relationships with narcissists to understand, let alone accept that the narcissist's behavior has nothing to do with the victim. They are responsible for their behavior, and we know— wrapping your head around this seems impossible. This is because if someone does anything bad to you, it is logical to conclude that they have a problem with you. In the world of the narcissist, however, this is not true, as humans do not matter. Narcissists usually are at war with themselves and you are just unlucky to be caught in the crossfire.

To a narcissist, you might be no one. The battle is internal, and their goal is to preserve themselves. Hence, even if it seems the narcissist is playing games with you and messing with your head, it is not so. To a narcissist, you are just a tool with which he can hurt himself or make himself feel good. This is hard to understand for many rational beings, because it involves a level of self-preservation so intense that other people become simply pawns. Even though, from an intellectual point of view, we claim to understand it and can explain it to others, emotionally, it will always be a mystery.

We consider the hurt from a narcissist as personal

because we examine the motive from our personal perspective. As a result, no matter what, the motive and hurt will be personal to you, and not the narcissist. Why will anyone want to hurt another person? Because deep down inside of them, there is hurt.

The narcissist is aware that you have not done anything to hurt or upset him. However, they see you as a representation of their failure. They have hurt and hatred rooted in their personality, and they know it. Even though narcissists might seem like sadists, they are not in reality. This is because sadists derive enjoyment from the pain and torture they inflict on their victim. Thus, for the torture to work on them, their victim must be thinking and feeling. Narcissists, however, are not wired this way. The pleasure comes from them, rather than from others. Hurting others makes them feel good, since it takes the pressure off of them.

This relationship can be likened to a person punching a bag. The "feel-good" feeling comes when you get a chance to blow off steam, not because you hurt the bag. The bag cannot feel the punches.

This points to the fact that a narcissist does not perceive humans the way other normal and sane people do.

Normal people see others as individuals with needs, desires, wishes, motivations, feelings, wants, likes, dislikes, goals, etc. To a narcissist, however, all of this does not make sense—and neither does he care. This is to tell you the extent of how emotionless a narcissist can be. You only matter to a narcissist as long as they can use you—that is all, nothing else matters. Not only does it not matter, he neither recognizes nor acknowledges it. This is why trying to make a narcissist see things from your point of view is a futile effort.

Considering all that has been explained above, it is not surprising that, to a narcissist, his behaviors are not abuse. This is due to the nature of the dysfunction of a narcissist. Truly, a narcissist is under constant attack, even though it is internal. This is why a narcissist can't consider himself as being an abuser, but a victim.

Abuse, to a narcissist, could be termed "cooling off" or "blowing off steam." This makes sense since abuse acknowledges the deliberate hurting of others, while blowing off steam does not in any way. It only has to do with the narcissist and his feelings and problems. This makes sense, because that is how they see things. No matter how many punches you throw at a punching bag, you cannot abuse it. Hence, the narcissist truly is not out to get or destroy you, since you are not human (to them). Rather, they care only about protecting themselves. This is shocking and even unbelievable to a rational human being, but this is how the narcissist is wired.

Note that this is only to give you a glimpse of the angle the narcissist is coming from. This is not to excuse or justify their behavior as not abusive; by all means, it is. The narcissist's motives do not matter, because the end result is the same. They are completely self-absorbed, abusive, and manipulative.

Still, this is a good foundation to understand them and their behavior. It can give you a solid grasp of how to handle them better. The idea behind this is not to see the narcissist as the problem, but that deep down inside of the narcissist, something is fundamentally wrong which controls his behavior. This can help you get closure and also realize that it is not about the narcissist, hence, they need to let go and move to a better, healthier, and happier life.

How to Confront a Narcissist in Their Behavior

What is the worst that can happen if you confront a narcissist? Will all hell let loose if you confront him? To really answer this, we need to examine the personality of the parties involved, as well as the circumstances. However, if you do want to confront a narcissist, you need to be clear on what you hope to achieve.

What do you want from this confrontation?

If you have your facts right and you are confident that your partner is a narcissist, you might be tempted to confront them. The sad part, however, is that it is a futile effort. This is because you will be disappointed if you think confronting the narcissist with the information of how they have made your life a living hell will make him change. You might think they would be remorseful or sorry, but it does not work that way.

This is because the emotional capacity of the narcissist is highly underdeveloped. As a result, they cannot understand or process this information, let alone accept the fact that they are not perfect. As a result, a narcissist is not equipped with the ability to search inside his soul and find out the truth.

With the above in mind, before you map out tactics to

confront the narcissist, be sure you know what you want from the interaction. If your expectation is fair treatment, equality, and some sense of acceptance in your relationship, it is better you move on. This is because there is little chance of success, and even if you have some, it will be minute, which comes with excessive investment in terms of time and effort.

If you are, however, in a position where moving on is difficult, then you need to arm yourself with useful tactics to make your confrontation fruitful.

Narcissist Reaction to Confrontation

When you confront a narcissist, their default reaction is rage or denial. The narcissist might deny everything, throw tantrums, say you are blowing things out of proportion, and eventually play the victim. Also, expect to have the narcissist turn everything around on you. For instance, if you confront them about spending too much time with the opposite sex, they may say you are too suspicious and do not trust them. If you decide to cope with this treatment, the following steps will help you confront them. However, hoping for any positive turnaround is an illusion. It will only end up setting you up for more pain and disappointment.

When confronting a narcissist, be prepared for the narcissist rage. The rage is their response to the injury that your criticism and disagreement inflicts on their self-esteem. They become enraged because they accept themselves as perfect, without flaws. To a narcissist, a slight disagreement or objection is humiliation. This is why they overreact, become defensive and aggressive, and attack the source of the injury. The person, in turn, suffers with criticism and serious downgrading. They believe in getting even, and if they cannot get even, they will lash out strongly at you in a bid to lessen the impact of the damage to their esteem.

How to Confront?

Sam Vaknin, a self-proclaimed narcissist, advises that the best way is to leave or threaten to leave a narcissist. The threat does not have to be conditional. If they yell at you, yell back at them, slam the door, and be insistent. This will give him a taste of his own medicine.

One of a narcissist's worst nightmares is abandonment. It stands above everything else the narcissist fears. This is why he begins to dread getting emotionally attached to another person. As a result, he misbehaves, acts cruel, and distances himself emotionally from the relationship. Eventually, the abandonment that he so terribly fears comes upon him.

This is the key to confronting a narcissist. Should he give an angry outburst, rage back at him, as well. This rekindles his worst nightmare—abandonment—which makes him come to his senses and he will retreat.

Bear in mind that for you to be successful in confronting a narcissist, you need to be strong. Alongside that, you need to have a good self-esteem and firmly believe you are an individual with rights—you do not deserve such cruel treatments.

How to Protect Yourself from a Narcissist

With an estimation that narcissists make up around 1% of the general population, there is a chance you will come across someone with Narcissistic Personality Disorder in your lifetime. Starting such a relation, however, comes with grave consequences Just like a fish is lured into a bait and pays later with her life, a narcissist lures seemingly innocent people with their charming and romantic behavior. Even though you might not pay with your life, you have a lot to lose.

This is why a good defense strategy is to learn how to protect yourself from such individuals. This revolves around training yourself to spot the red flags these individuals emit. In other words, it takes being able to see past their charming personality and captivating talk.

In the same way, it is important to protect yourself from falling prey to another narcissist if you recently ended a relationship with one. This involves developing and restoring your core self. In other words, you need to cultivate the healthy practice of connecting to your life. It is about coming up with authentic and healthy ways of relating with yourself, such that what attracted you to the narcissist is gone.

Know Who a Narcissist is

This is the first step in knowing how to protect yourself from a narcissist. You cannot keep yourself away from what you do not know. This is where many people miss it. They have such faith in the goodness of man in general that it is impossible for them to accept that some people could be so callous, mean, and emotionless.

Many people are also fond of giving strangers the benefit of the doubt. However, equipping yourself with the idea of who a narcissist is and how they behave can go a long way in saving yourself months, years, or even a lifetime of misery.

If you have come this far with this manual, I believe you already have an idea of the kind of person a narcissist is. As a summary, keep an eye out for red flags like your partner constantly feeling like they are better than everyone else, with a conviction that they cannot be wrong; someone who takes excessive pride in their accomplishments; reveals a desperate need for admiration; or behaves in a cocky, patronizing, demanding, and self-absorbed manner.

Connect to Your Mind and Body

To protect yourself from a narcissist, you need to be happy and comfortable with yourself. This involves knowing what you want, what you want to be, how you want others to perceive you, and having access to your inner resources. This authenticity allows them respond with wisdom to all the tactics of the narcissist, rather than with fear.

Narcissist do not like the truth and people in tune with their inner being is a strong repellant to them. Hence, to defeat a narcissist is not about the ability to argue and reason things out. By the time a narcissist employs cruel tactics like gaslighting, your ability to reason will be crushed. In fact, some narcissists love the challenge of conquering strong and passionate women.

Strive to Know Yourself

An authentic person has a lifelong mission of knowing and understanding themselves. This helps them understand others, which guides their life, relations, and interactions. This makes them happy and contented with life and all it has to offer, while striving to improve themselves. Connecting with yourself allows you to develop a unique understanding of yourself and others.

When you consider a narcissist, they cannot engage in normal conversation. If you have ever had deep conversations (hopes, dreams, fears, etc.) with a narcissist, with the hope that they will reason, love, and empathize with you, you are wrong. All he is interested in is information with which he can control and use against you with time.

With an authentic person, however, a narcissist is powerless. This is due to their inability to spot loopholes to prey on, to instill fear, gaslight, and manipulate. The narcissist detests being seen for who they really are. They do not like being seen as emotionally weak, because in their mind, showing love and being compassionate is for the weak.

Have a Strong Inner Sense of Control

True happiness comes from within, and authentic people know this. As a result, they can enjoy the peace and tranquility they seek. This gives them the capacity to detach their emotions from issues that they know are the narcissist's. They can deal with and control personal issues, and also separate these from the narcissists, irrespective of how the narcissist tries to manipulate them.

They are aware of the tactics the narcissist employs, so despite everything the narcissist does, they can relax and prevent upsetting emotions from springing up. This is not surprising, since it is normal for the narcissist to always try to make their partner panic. It is common for the narcissist to be stuck in a cycle of making their partner take the fall of all wrongdoings. For instance:

- Behaving like they are not receiving adequate love and attention

- Feel like it is their right to treat others badly

- Make others responsible for their own woes

- Expect to be treated as if they are special

A narcissist is not interested in healing and getting better. To them, this is for the weak, as they do not even believe anything is wrong with them. Hence, a real person will not be surprised by these behaviors and will not even expect improvement. As a result, they know that the best way to handle them is to keep their own emotions in check. In other words, they are not surprised each time the narcissist acts irrationally.

Many people are shocked and disturbed when the narcissist misbehaves, because they expect better. Yet, over time, their actions and behaviors have followed the same pattern—expecting an improvement is setting oneself up for disappointment. When the narcissist, however, sees that all his action has no effect on you, your fear system refuses to be activated, they are starved of what keeps them fulfilled. With time, they will let you be.

Make What Hurts and Makes You Vulnerable a Secret

Vulnerable emotions are part of what makes us human. It is vital to a balanced life and should only be shared with people you trust—not a narcissist. This is because emotions that make us vulnerable are important sources of power that make us human.

A narcissist's mindset and view of others around is way different from that of normal people. He might put up an act to show as if he cares about your problem, but he's gathering information about you. These are data that he will use to manipulate you, instill fear, confuse your thinking faculties, etc. In other words, to you, you feel you are pouring your heart to someone while the narcissist is nothing more than a scientist gathering data.

Stay Firm and Grounded

We all have an intuition that knows things even without much fact. People might call this gut or sixth senses. Your gut can warn you of dangers and give you strong feelings when you are trying to make a decision. Hence, if you meet someone and they appear too good to be true, listen to your gut.

Narcissist are charming, sometimes with charisma and an outgoing personality. This is often in a bid to bait unsuspecting people. If your sixth sense is warning you, draw the curtain.

When next you are with someone who makes you question your self-worth, remind yourself of how important and special you are. Make it a personal rule to take your time in getting to know someone. Do not be caught in the drama and do not feel compelled to explain your values life choices to the narcissist. Remember, they only care about getting you entangled in their web, to use you as a source for their evil whims.

How to Break Up With a Narcissist

Dating a narcissist is draining and exhausting. This is not surprising, because of their vain, manipulative, self-absorbed, competitive, and proud nature. To break up with a narcissist, you need to be well prepared. Bear in mind that rejection does not go well with a narcissist. as they are likely to view it as an attack and respond with strong backlash and hostility—no matter how careful you are.

In dealing with a narcissist, you need to be smart. A narcissist might not even attack you. On the contrary, he might break down, sob, and plead with the promise to change, appealing to your compassionate side not to sever the tie.

You might not be able to predict the narcissist reaction. However, it is important to take important steps to protect yourself and tactically end such a toxic relationship.

Before the Breakup

Breaking up with a narcissist is dealing a big blow to their pride. Hence, humiliation is not negotiable, if and when you reject a narcissist. As a result, prepare your mind for drama as they will likely try to turn the tables around, dominating the conversation.

The key here is limiting the time you spend on the breakup, and make sure it is done in the company of friends or loved ones. This makes the situation less dramatic.

During the Conversation

In breaking up with a narcissist, you need to outsmart them. This is not a time for honesty, because they will manipulate what you say and even use it against you.

This is not the time to rant about how they have made your life a living hell, or how they have ruined everything. Neither should you tell them how much they are suffocating you. Rather, tell them you are not good for each other, and the relationship is not working for either of you.

Assigning blame will not do any good here, as narcissists are good at playing defense when they feel at fault. The idea is to make the reason for the breakup as vague and general as possible. Keep the list of hurts and cons to yourself.

Having established this foundation, how do you go about severing the tie with your narcissist partner?

Steps in Breaking Up with a Narcissist

Reconnect With Long Lost Friends

There is a big chance that being with a narcissist has isolated you from your friends and loved ones. This could happen due to many reasons. Your partner might have tried to separate you from any support system you have. Your friends might have criticized your partner and relationship in the past, and you ended up staying away from them to limit the criticism.

You have got to mend these broken bridges, since you will need all the support you can get during and after the breakup. Their support is vital to get you through the breakup.

Clean Up Your Social Media Account

We admit, this is harsh but necessary to fast track your healing. The less reminders and associations of your narcissist partner you have, the less intense the impact of the breakup will be. Be ruthless about this, as it does not exclude their families. Get rid of them from your Facebook, LinkedIn, Instagram, Twitter, etc.

If you have any link or connection via a relation or friend, the narcissist can use this as a link back to your life. They can also use it as a means to make you jealous. Only keep friends you know and trust very well.

Sever the Tie Abruptly—No Long Goodbyes

To prevent unnecessary emotions, make the breakup clean, clear, and concise. Do not give room for explanation, hugs, arguments, or a chance for them to explain their behavior or cajole you thinking you can make it work. The longer you tarry, the more chances the narcissist has to twist facts and try to convince you are making a huge mistake.

Always Remind Yourself Why You Are Breaking Up

Breaking up with a sane person is hard in itself. But breaking up with a narcissist is harder, because you are leaving injured with a battered self-esteem. After the relief of getting hold of your life, you need to rejoice in the opportunity to pick yourself up and rebuild yourself. A constant reminder of why the relationship is unhealthy for you is necessary to keep you going.

Being with a narcissist is draining. They make mountains out of molehills. Gradually, they sap you of your self-esteem. They act cold in a bid to make you struggle for their love. Reflect on every curse word, how they made you feel worthless and sad, and the misery they caused you.

Your friends can be of terrific help in reminding you why you are better off without the narcissist. I bet they remember every time you reached out to them because of how your ex treated you. The knowledge of why you should regain your freedom will keep you going.

Prepare for Backlash

You just rejected a narcissist—do not expect them to let it go easily. Hence, you need to prepare for various kind of fallout. They will try all means to bring you down, even if it means bad-mouthing you to family and friends. They will try to tarnish your reputation in all ways.

The best strategy is to prepare yourself and your loved ones. Let them know you are ending the relationship and the tendency of your ex to come back at you. Even if there will not be a fallout, it is good not to be caught unawares.

Be Prepared for Begging and Pleading

If you are the one that initiated the breakup, what a bold decision! However, you need to brace up for impact. Losing does not go over well with a narcissist; hence, they will do all in their capacity to make sure their supply is intact, even if it involves begging.

As a result, there will be all form of promises to turn over a new leaf. Expect acts of kindness, doing things you have wanted them to do, all in an effort to try to get you reconsider. They might go as far as telling you that you are lost without them.

Their tactic is to instill fear in you, with the hope that you will reconsider. Beware, and stand your ground.

Have a Solid No-Contact Rule

No contact is as simple as it sounds—get them to back off. If they want to be violent, go for a restraining order. But this is not about physical contact alone. Block every avenue with which they can reach out to you, which involves getting rid of them from your social media accounts and blocking their number. It is good to do this as soon as possible, to block every avenue for them to return.

Bear in mind that they will try all means to make contact. And when they do, they know just the right words to say to get you reconsider. This is why you need to be brutal. If you cannot stand the various emotions that will fly around when you confront them with breakup, do it via text.

Expect Them to Move on Fast, and Rub it in Your Face

If you are dealing with a narcissist, they will not need time to heal from the breakup. Think about it: they never loved you in the first place. All through the relationship, they were mostly absent and insincere. If they did truly care about you, they would not treat you like trash. To a narcissist, you are just a source to fuel their ego and help boost their self-esteem. After the breakup, if you are resilient enough to turn down all their pleading and advances, their next move is to look for their next victim to prey on.

Also, a narcissist might already have an exit strategy, should the present relationship fail. Hence, once you pull the plug, they move on to their next target.

Realize You Are Mourning What You Never Had

I will not sugarcoat things and tell you the breakup will be easy. No, it will not. You will feel sad, dejected, full of regret, anxious, etc. It is all part of the grieving process. However, you can take solace in the fact that what you had was not real. You didn't lose a relationship—you lost your self-esteem and confidence, and you lost a toxic person that was out to destroy you. Many questions and thoughts will run through your mind, such as:

- How could I be so stupid to fall in love with him?

- How did he get away with manipulating me for so long?

- Why couldn't I see through the lies?

You will want to beat yourself up as you ruminate through the whole thing. Bear in mind, it was never your fault. Narcissists are skilled at pretending and manipulating you to see them as all you want in a partner. They are masters of deception and, just like a chameleon, they will blend in. You are not to blame for not seeing him for who he really is.

What to Expect After Breaking Up With a Narcissist

When you break up with a narcissist, the battle is not over. In fact, we know that being in a relationship with a narcissist is awful. However, breaking up with one is even worse. This section will guide you on what to expect when you break up with a narcissist.

Narcissist do not Throw in the Towel Easily

In other words, do not expect a narcissist to go down without a fight. In fact, the breakup period might be the time you will see them at their worst. Expect them to come hard at you with various tactics, all in bid to manipulate and instill fear.

The key is to be strategic, as well, and let go of your emotions. This will protect you from any psychological fallout. We also recommend having someone who understands the mind of a narcissist. If you are married, for instance, it is recommended you go for a lawyer that has handled divorce cases involving a narcissistic spouse.

Narcissist do not Believe in Losing

Divorce and breakup is so traumatic that no one wins. However, the ability of the parties involved to come to a fair agreement could help soften the blow. If you are with a narcissist, however, nothing you can come up with will be just. They do not like to back down, as negotiation or mediation is a sign of weakness, a defeat they are not ready to accept.

They want to be right and will do anything to prove it, even if it means telling a lie. They do not mind how much they hurt or damage you in the process, as long as they are able to save face and get what they want.

They do not Mind Playing Dirty

If you are going through a divorce, they do not mind exposing your deep, dark secrets, even in the courtroom. All the things you shared in confidence will be used against you. He will also cook things up to make you appear like the bad guy before the judge.

A narcissist's desire to win against all odds trumps everything. Hence, they do not mind who gets hurt in the process. Expect him to bad-mouth you to your friends, family, colleagues, loved ones, and anyone that cares to listen.

They Will Even Try to Gaslight You

One of the inherent traits of a narcissist is that they like playing the victim. They have the ability to confuse you until they become the victim and even make you feel bad for trying to sever your ties with them.

And if you are compelled to bare your mind before him (which is a terrible, terrible idea), they will find a way of bringing everything back to you, making you the cause of their behavior and misfortune.

Take this as a warning and do not fall for this tactic. You can render him powerless by focusing on the issues at hand, irrespective of whatever he says. This is part of why we advise minimizing communication during the breakup. If there are kids involved, then discuss custody and visitation before you sever all forms of communication. Get rid of every chance to expose yourself to your partner's abuse.

They Will Not Give up Without a Fight

There is a huge chance they will refuse all forms of negotiation during the process, especially if it is a divorce. This is because, to a narcissist, nothing else is accepted, except that they win. Negotiation, in a narcissist's mind, is a form of defeat; hence, not accepted.

So, you likely have joint assets or kids in which you have to decide on custody and support arrangements—expect them not to make things easy. They will fight, drag, humiliate you, etc.

Breaking up with normal and sane people in itself is hard. However, when it is with a narcissistic partner, it is harder. As a result, you'll need all the help and preparation you can get to make the process smooth. This chapter has provided detailed information on how to things easier, irrespective of all the tantrums and backlash of the narcissist. With determination, strength, and courage, you can come out strong.

Chapter 4: Recommended Activities for Recovery

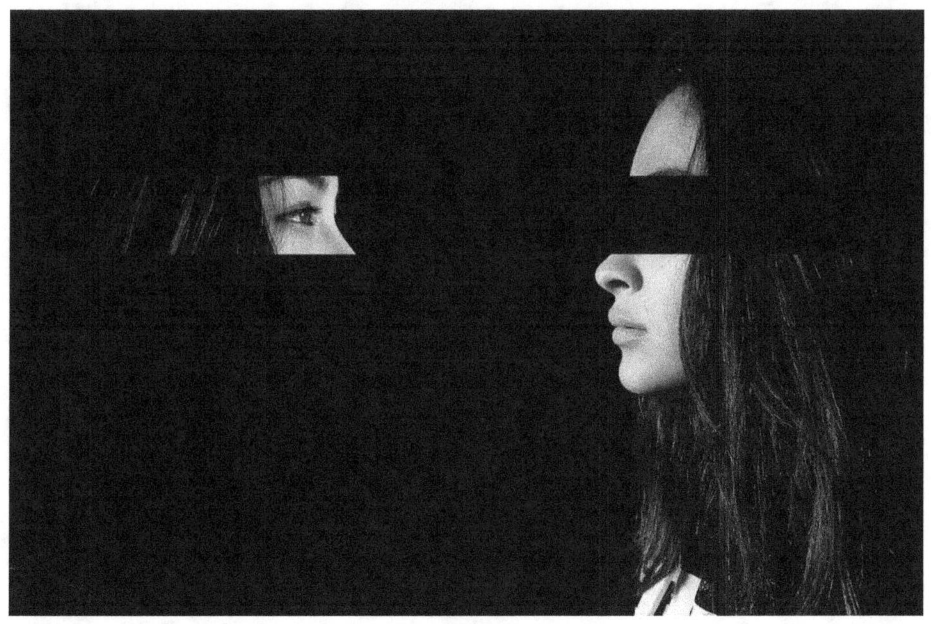

Leaving a toxic relationship with a narcissist is not a simple process. After finding the courage to end the relationship, you need to take steps to recover and get your sanity back. This is due to the fact that there will be a devastating effect on your psychological health. As a result, victims might experience nightmares, depression, anxiety, dissociation, recurring flashbacks, low self-esteem, etc. And if you are unlucky to have had a fairly long relationship with the narcissist, you might have developed an intense trauma bond due to the incessant cycle of abuse.

As a result, you need to engage in helpful activities to recover from the trauma. You need to take care of yourself in every positive way possible. This way, you can regain your mind, spirit, and body after the abuse.

This chapter focuses on practical real-life steps you can implement to end self-sabotaging habits, reinforce positive self-esteem, and protect your core values.

Interviewing Yourself

We are constantly talking to ourselves throughout our waking moments, and the majority of this inner self-talk is a reflection of how valuable we consider ourselves to be. Our self-talk is largely shaped by the things we were told about ourselves from childhood, and our life experiences while growing up. It can also be shaped by the experiences we have in our relationships as adults. Staying in an abusive relationship can make our inner self-talk predominantly negative. Worse still, we may not notice, because this negative way of conversing inwardly has become so habituated and automatic that it feels normal.

Part of the recovery process from a narcissist's abuse requires that your self-talk becomes predominantly positive, loving, supportive, and kind. Practice the following exercises to quiet down negative self-talk so that you can habituate positive self-talk.

Thought Awareness Exercise

At several intervals during the day, catch yourself thinking about yourself and notice what the contents of your thoughts are.

Do not judge the thought as bad or good. Simply observe them the way you observe your breath.

Write down a brief statement that captures what those thoughts are. For example, "I am thinking about how changing my mind will make everyone feel disappointed in me."

Next, write down as many statements as you can that question the thought. This step challenges your thinking patterns and helps you turn down the volume of the negativity in your head. Using the example above, you can question the thought by writing, "*How do I know that everyone will feel disappointed if I change my mind?*" This question can lead to an answer such as, "*Since the new people in my life are supportive of me, they will understand that changing my mind will be beneficial to me.*"

The more times in a day you can do this, the better your chances will be of diminishing thoughts that are not supportive of you.

Periodic Self-Interview

Attempting to keep track of your every thought can make you miss the fun of living. To ease the process of checkmating your negative self-talk, you can set timers at several intervals throughout your day to ask yourself some questions about your self-talk. When the timer goes off, ask yourself the following questions:

What were my inner conversations for the past 30 minutes, one hour, or whatever time interval you used for your reminder?

What was the tone of your inner self-talk in the past period? Is it reassuring, kind, and supportive, or harsh, demeaning, and scalding? Would you speak to a dear friend this way?

When you are stressed or anxious, try and ask yourself what the content of your self-talk is. The simple act of noticing that you are experiencing an anxious moment is a huge win for you, because it will make you take it easy on yourself and not judge yourself harshly.

Reinvigorating Your Sense of Perception

A relationship with a narcissist changes your perception of yourself. But it doesn't happen overnight. It is not a demolition process—instead, it is a deconstruction process. For example, some narcissists don't put you down directly, but they do so in the guise of being realistic and implying that you can't succeed. They do this until you can't seem to react for yourself without thinking about what they would say or do, bringing you to the point where your perceptions about yourself became heavily thwarted. This took a lot of time and constant chipping away at your self-esteem. Reversing this perception about yourself is also going to be a process—one that involves a gradual reconstruction of what has been de-constructed.

Below are some practical exercises that can reinvigorate your sense of perception about yourself. Keep in mind that this process is a slow and continuous one. Do not expect to wake up tomorrow with a completely different perception about yourself. Such huge quantum jumps are not sustainable.

Do Something You Were Told You Can't Do

It doesn't matter if it is a career choice, a hobby, or some experience you've always wanted to explore—go ahead and do it. This is how you've always wanted to live, and no one should tell you what you can or cannot do. However, make sure that whatever you choose to do should be because you thoroughly enjoy doing it or you really want to experience it, and not out of spite for the abusive partner (or ex-partner). Acting out of spite means that the narcissist still has control over you. Let your choices be completely yours.

Reconnect with Positive People and Ideas

The way you perceive yourself is a function of the ideas you hold about yourself. Your ideas are built from what you hear others say about you and the ideas you entertain about yourself. Positive people uphold ideas and thoughts that are supportive of you and can rebuild a positive perspective about yourself.

Readjust Your Perspective with This Questionnaire

Take some time to honestly fill out this questionnaire and review your answers at frequent intervals. The goal of this is to help you see how beneficial your leaving an abusive or narcissist relationship is. This will reinforce your stance and view.

These are the top three things I stand to gain by quitting this relationship: (List them down and add to the list anytime you think of something new.)

Apart from me, the following people will benefit if I leave this relationship: (Write down each of their names— friends, children, etc.)

In the next six months, I would like to see myself: (Write down the things you would like to achieve, experience, and feel that reflect the positive way you want to see yourself.)

When I have stayed away from all forms of contact and communication with the abusive person, I will reward myself with: (Write down what you'll gift yourself, how you'll celebrate, or how you will treat yourself nicely.)

Assuming I have only six months left to live, I would: (Write down all the exciting things you've always wanted to do and begin to do them now.)

Group Therapy

If you are struggling to pick yourself up after quitting a narcissist relationship, group therapy is a recommended healing approach. The years you have spent with the narcissist will have dealt a significant blow on your self-esteem. You are always anxious and you always feel powerless, but you can be helped. After leaving an abusive partner, often, they've made you lose faith in yourself such that trusting another person becomes hard.

For you to recover from a narcissist's abuse, you need all the help you can get. The relationship has drained you so much that even though you know there is more to life, you are confused on how to go about it. Some people resort to drinking, drugs, sex, etc., in a bid to disguise their pain. This, however, does not bring true transformation.

In subjecting yourself to group therapy, you need an effective approach that will bring a complete turnaround in your life. This transformation can be possible without making you relive painful traumas. How will group therapy help you?

- It can help you break free of your addiction to your narcissistic partner, allowing you to go on living on your terms without him controlling you subconsciously.

- Get rid of abuse symptoms, no matter how long you have been abused.

- Live free of the trauma and symptoms of PTSD that came with the abuse.

- Be strengthened to let go of toxic shame and everything that happened to you.

- Believe in yourself again and have faith in the future, with renewed strength and hope to face life again.

- Develop, or get back your self-love and self-confidence.

I am sure there are dozens or hundreds of therapy groups around. However, you want to be sure the therapy you choose will help you get your life in order. As a result, you need to make sure that group therapy will help you achieve many things. Here are some things you should look for before subscribing to a group therapy session:

- Ability to help you release pain, the feeling of abuse and its trauma

- Let go of the false illusion that the narcissist is your whole world

- Ability to help you forgive yourself for falling for the narcissist's trap and embrace life all over again

- Let go of the pain of betrayal from the person you trusted

- Release your narcissist partner and your quest to make them pay for all they made you live through

- Be free from the fear of the narcissist and what he might do next

- Embrace your freedom

You will likely need more than coaching or talk therapy to recover after the abuse. What you want is an encompassing program that will bring an all-round transformation

Dialectical Behavior Therapy (DBT)

Developed in 1980, Dialectical Behavior Therapy (DBT) is a form of cognitive-behavioral psychotherapy that is used to treat borderline personality disorder. Since its development, however, it has been used to treat other types of mental health disorders, including post-traumatic stress disorder. This is common to victims of narcissistic abuse; hence, it can be of great help.

DBT revolves around the fact that some people can give an intense reaction towards some emotional situations, commonly with family, friends, and romantic partners. DBT explains that in some emotional situations, some people give a stronger reaction than the average person. Besides that, it takes a whole lot of time for these people to calm down and return to baseline levels.

As a result of the abuse of being in a narcissistic relationship, there might be some psychological effects—for instance, extreme emotional swings, trauma, and an intense surge of emotions. Very few people understand this; hence, there might not be an effective coping mechanism.

DBT uses various techniques to help patients—one of such is validation. When you leave a narcissist relationship, there might be distress at the thought of being alone and losing your partner. This technique helps victims embrace the change that comes with leaving such a relationship.

Components of Dialectical Behavior Therapy

I. **Support-Oriented:** This seeks to identify a person's strength and build on it. With this, the person will feel good about themselves and their overall life. This can help build the self-esteem that has been sapped gradually during the relationship.

II. **Cognitive-Based:** This seeks thought, ideas, assumptions, and beliefs that make life hard. "If I raise my voice, I am a horrible person." "I have to please everyone around me." On identifying these thoughts, DBT helps suggest alternative thinking patterns that are acceptable." Everyone gets angry and raises their voice, and it is a normal emotion." "I do not have to please everyone, because that is impossible."

III.   **Collaborative:** DBT encourages clients to express issues in their relationship with their therapist. There will be homework, role-play, suggested ways of interacting with others, etc. There will be practice suggestions to help calm the nerves when upset. The therapist works with the client to learn, apply, and master these.

The Four Skill Modules

DBT skill training revolves around four modules: core mindfulness, distress tolerance, emotion regulation, and interpersonal effectiveness. They are structured mainly to help people manage their emotions, thoughts, behaviors, and reactions. It was designed with the aim of helping people in chaotic or abusive relationships, in which narcissistic relationships fit in perfectly.

Core mindfulness helps the victim focus on their mind. With distress tolerance, the client is able to accept, judge and evaluate their circumstances and also develop crisis survival skills. This helps limit their chance of developing problematic behavior. With emotion regulation, the client learns to recognize and label present emotions, know what stops the current emotions from changing, suppress emotional reactivity, and boost positive emotions, etc. Interpersonal Effectiveness skills teach effective and polite strategies for coping with conflict, asking for what you need, and saying no without feeling guilty.

Core Mindfulness Skills

The mindfulness skills adopted in DBT help patients focus on the present. In other words, clients learn how to focus on what is happening currently and accept it in a calm and peaceful way. It was adapted from the eastern spiritual traditions. People can bring themselves to the present and concentrate on what they need to care for themselves. This technique helps patients deal with intense emotions wisely, rather than reacting destructively.

Interpersonal Effectiveness Skills

This helps people know and realize what they want in their relationships. Not only that, they will learn effective strategies of dealing and relating with others in a bid to reach these goals. Some of the strategies thought include respecting themselves and the other person, learning to express themselves without fear or coming off as arrogant, and relating with difficult people, as well as the ability to object to people without feeling guilty.

Distress Tolerance

There are many treatments for mental health that focus on tackling distressing events with the aim of providing solutions. They have left out the place of accepting, learning to live with, and finding meaning with distress. The aim of this module, however, is to help patients learn how to bear the pain.

Victims will learn to accept the situation, without judgment and evaluation of the circumstance. In other words, you are not at fault for attracting a narcissist. The relationship already happened, and you were a victim. Rather, you will learn helpful skills that can help you survive the aftermath of this relationship. Here, there are four strategies for crisis survival: distracting, self-soothing, improving the moment, and considering the pros and cons.

Emotion Regulation

After ending a narcissistic relationship, you cannot remain the same. There will surely be a surge of intense emotion. You will be angry, frustrated, filled with regrets, anxious, afraid, hurt, and even depressed. This is why learning to regulate these emotions come in. Emotion regulation will help patients to:

- Recognize and distinguish the right emotions

- Know what stops emotions from changing

- Boost positive emotions

- Encourage awareness of current emotions

- Make the best use of distress tolerance techniques

Meditation

Narcissistic relationships can leave victims severely traumatized. Trauma affects humans negatively, such that parts of the brain that handle learning, memory, focus, emotional regulation, planning, etc. lose coordination. However, some of the stress from the separation can be alleviated through meditation. Meditation has been shown to be of tremendous benefit to the parts of the brain that suffers this trauma, like the amygdala, hippocampus, and the prefrontal cortex. (Lazar, 2016).

With meditation, survivors can take control of their lives. As a result of the wonderful effect of meditation on the brain, it can help survivors embrace reality and restructure their brain such that they are empowered, not under the influence of the trauma.

With meditation, you can be in control of your emotions instead of allowing them to control you. It can help you consider your options and really make sense of what you want to do before you do it. Hence, you learn to carefully examine whatever emotions you have before acting impulsively. Even if you are considering the urge to reach out to your ex, meditation helps you consider the pros and cons as well as other alternatives. With meditation, you can soothe the impact of the trauma.

The effect of meditation to heal after breaking up with a narcissist cannot be overemphasized. The best part about this practice, however, is that you might not have to dedicate hours before reaping the benefits.

How to Practice Brief Meditation

If you have enough time to dedicate to meditation, it will be very effective in soothing your wounds. However, the problem for many people is finding the time to meditate. When you think about everything demanding for your attention, planning time to meditate might not come easy. This is why we recommend three minutes or less. The advantage of this is that you can do it anywhere, and many times a day, even on your busiest day

How to Go About Brief Meditation

Find a comfortable position to sit down—it could be on a chair, stool, or on the bare floor. This is not rigid; the idea is to be comfortable, without any part of the body tensed. Make sure your body parts are all free: your hands could be on your lap, faced up or free sideways. Do whatever feels natural and follow the following steps:

I.   *Concentrate on Your Breath*: Direct your focus to your breath as it passes through and leaves your nostril. Pay attention to the up and down movement of your abdomen as the air fills and leaves your stomach.

II.   *Scan Your Body: Consider* each part of your body separately and search for any tension. Massage your wrist as you imagine your breath soothing this tension.

III. *Observe Your Thoughts:* Without judging, think about what is going on in your mind. Carefully bring your mind back to a place of rest.

IV.   *Embrace Your Feelings:* Emotions are not part of you; they come and go. This is why it is recommended that you accept your emotions when you are dealing with trauma.

V.   *Watch*: Chose an object and lock your gaze intently. It could be a butterfly, a flowing river, a flower swaying with the wind, etc.

VI.   *Choose a Mantra:* A mantra, in this case, is anything that works for you. It could be "I am free," "I am whole," "I am perfect," etc. The idea is to heal your subconscious of any psychological trauma the abuser might have caused.

VII. *Reach Out and Touch:* We recommend having a

bead or a hand band. Whenever you see the bead or the hand band, consider it a trigger to bring your mind to a calm state of rest.

Examples of How to Practice Brief Meditations

I. *Employ Traffic Lights:* If you drive or move around with public taxis or bus, you can employ traffic signals. Traffic signals can help bring your thoughts to a peaceful state where you can breathe easier.

II. *While You Walk:* As you trek to the grocery store across the neighborhood, focus on your footsteps and meditate. If you have time to jog or use the treadmill, meditate for a couple of minutes as you do so.

III. *Bond with Your Kids:* Even your kids or pets could benefit from meditation—have fun and spend this meaningful time together. Sing together, employ visualization, or you can take a walk with your kids or pets.

IV. *Line Up:* The next time you are waiting in a queue for movie tickets or a cup of coffee, use that time to meditate. All you need to do is focus on your breath.

V.   *Wash Mindfully*: The next time you have a shower, be sure to apply every sponge stroke mindfully. Focus on the stoking process and use it to bring order to your thoughts.

Meditation is one of the simplest, healthiest, and least expensive responses to stress. No matter how traumatized you are, meditation can help lessen the blow of your breakup. There are guided meditation scripts online and on YouTube that can be of tremendous help.

Cognitive Behavioral Therapy (CBT)

Popularly known as CBT, this is a form of therapy that examines the influence of our thoughts on our behaviors. In other words, it helps people, including victims of narcissistic abuse, to discover how their thoughts, attitudes and beliefs affect their disposition to life. The goal of CBT is to help patients develop healthy and positive coping mechanisms for difficult life situations.

Cognitive Behavioral Therapy helps individuals focus on what is happening at the moment. When this is identified, the patient can learn positive coping mechanisms by examining and challenging such emotions.

How Cognitive Behavioral Therapy Works

After breaking up with a narcissist, the victim might experience flashbacks, which could result in trauma and other psychological problems. With CBT, victims can learn to understand and deal with these destructive thoughts such that they do not traumatize them again.

This often involves the joint collaboration of the patient and therapy to analyze the situation. After this, they can come up with a treatment plan that will help change such challenging thoughts and feelings. Here are some of the aims of CBT:

- Helps victims recognize thoughts that are not healthy

- Improves their self confidence

- Teaches healthy coping mechanisms in stressful situations

- Teaches how to avoid surges of emotion in distressing situations

Compared to other forms of therapy, cognitive behavioral therapy is brief. The initial phase of CBT will be dedicated to examining the abusive relationship that just ended. There will be sections to address the trauma and psychological effects of the abuse on the victim. For instance, you might tend to become a people pleaser, walking on eggshells and lacking confidence as an aftermath of the situation. CBT can help unlearn destructive habits with specific techniques, and also recommends healthy alternatives.

Being in an abusive relationship for a long time has a tarnishing effect on one's self-esteem. CBT will help the victim analyze the circumstances where their self-esteem was battered. This is essential to the victim regaining their sanity and reducing the risk of future issues. CBT can also help victims understand the tactics with which the narcissist wrecked their self-esteem. All the lies, manipulations, and abusive behaviors, etc., will be examined and the therapist can help the victim see why they should stop believing them.

Part of the aim of a CBT session is to develop coping skills to reduce the effect of the trauma that follows the breakup. CBT will also help you accept that you were not responsible for your abusive partner's behavior. This way, you are able to improve your self-esteem until it's easier to think about putting yourself out there for a better relationship. Additionally, you stop thinking less of yourself and also believe in your ability to have a meaningful relationship.

In Conclusion

The damage that an abusive relationship causes is extensive. This is why you need to get creative and smart in seeking help after the breakup. We have presented many recommended activities for recovery for you to consider which works best for you.

Chapter 5: Alternative Healing Methods Explained

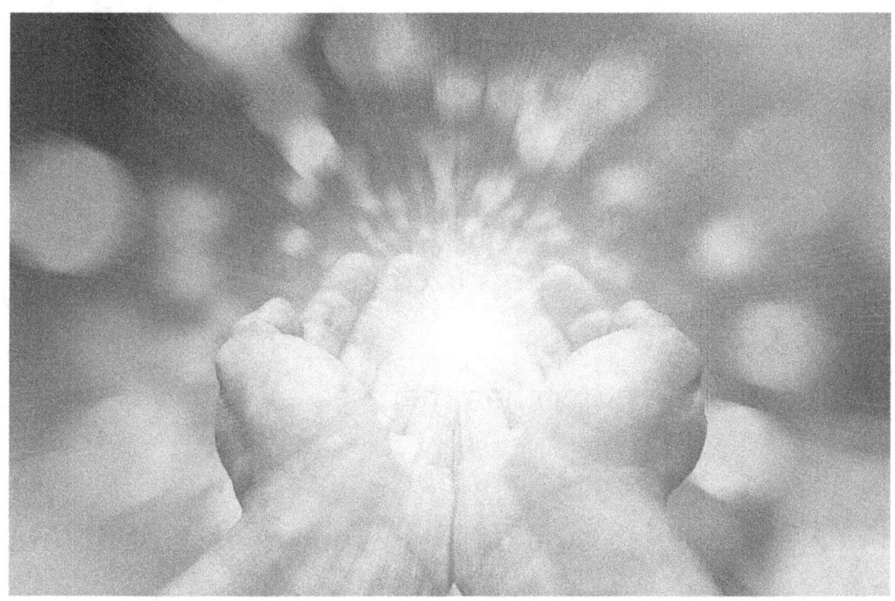

There are many helpful and potent healing methods you can use to get your life in order after leaving an abusive relationship. Your well-being is important, so be sure to embrace every opportunity you have to heal. If you would like an overhaul of your spirit, soul, mind, and body, the following proven healing techniques can be of significant help.

Eye-Movement Desensitization and Reprocessing (EMDR) Therapy for Narcissist Abuse Recovery

If you need therapy to reduce the physiological distress that comes with traumatic memories, like those from an abusive relationship, EMDR is a good option. This is because it can reduce or even completely eliminate the after-effect of such recollections. This happens by directing the attention, and the memory, at something else—something other than themselves.

Unlike CBT and other forms of therapy, you will not have to talk about what is going on in your mind. Rather, this relies on stimulating the brain using the immediate surroundings. Hence, EMDR tries to alter any emotions that arise months or weeks after an occurrence when they tap in to some part of their brain. These are parts of the brain that bring about such emotions when they reflect.

EMDR is unique and has been proven to be effective, because victims do not need many sessions before improvement begins. When the eyes move rapidly, it helps open up the brain neural network. This allows memories to be processed uniquely in a safe and healthy environment, besides the one responsible for the trauma. The idea is to replace these memories with empowering thoughts and feelings. The end game is to ensure that such memories do not create anxiety, fear, hatred, depression, and other symptoms of Post-Traumatic Stress Disorder that comes from an abuse. As a result, the person is free to embrace life and all it has, even to start a new relationship without fear.

Victims of narcissistic relationships are characterized by tons of negative memories and abuse that can be sexual, verbal, emotional, or physical.

While in an EMDR therapy section, the victim will have to access and think about one of the memories of such abusive episodes. This happens while they keep their eye on an external stimuli for a couple of seconds.

The victim does not focus on the negative alone. This is done alongside a focus on positive affirmations, a discussion, or fresh thoughts. During the session, there are many things that can happen to such negative memories, for instance:

- The detail might begin to die down.
- The experience might feel less overwhelming.

- Their emotional reaction to the memory might be less encompassing.

- The person might even have a different reaction to such memory, for instance, humor for the abuser.

This happens because there is a "reconfiguration" of the brain that allows the person in therapy to view the event differently. One of the ways EMDR helps victim is that the significance of the trauma fades. This puts them in control of their memory and emotions.

EMDR and Victims of Narcissistic Abuse

Abuse comes in various forms. When many people think of abuse, they imagine name calling, humiliation, physical harm, emotional shattering, etc.

When it comes to narcissistic abuse, however, the above is not enough to illustrate it. This is because the damage done by a narcissist cannot be expressed in terms of the traditional ways people consider abuse.

This is not to say that a narcissistic abuser will not do the above. There is a significant probability that they will. But underneath this is a devious means in which they control, harm and disorient their victim, through deception, brainwashing, gaslighting, etc.

Narcissists are not honest about themselves, their intentions, or their past experiences. You can never really get to know them, as they will not be straight with their emotions, their motivations, and what is going on in their mind. You will not even know when they are telling the truth. They were never really present in the relationship, as they blocked every avenue for you to get to know them.

They are fond of using deception to brainwash their victims. As a result, the relationship is characterized by psychological and intense forms of abuse that go beyond the normal forms. There are times the narcissist could use other people to manipulate you. Both of you might agree on a rule, but the narcissist will break such boundaries at will. Narcissists also do things covertly—in other words, there might not be any memory to associate such event with.

Much of the damage the victim experiences happens in the dark. If this abuse occurs over a long term, it can result in brain damage. This is because it keeps the amygdala in a state of anxiety. This is the typical state in which most narcissist abuse victims find themselves. This is why EMDR proves to be very useful, as it tries to correct the brain damage caused by the abuse.

In summary, EMDR therapy employs dual-attention stimulus to change the effect of trauma in the body. This therapy uses tapping, tactile stimulation, headphones, or eye movement to access the part of the brain that processes information. This lessens the effect of the trauma such that you will be able to cope without negative emotional reaction.

Emotional Freedom Technique

Another effective strategy to help lessen the traumatizing effects of narcissistic abuse is emotional freedom technique. It is simple, free, and can be done without a therapist, in the comfort of your home. You can also work with a skilled EFT therapist or a friend to help you get through the trauma.

ETF, also known as tapping involves a technique in which all patients have to do is tap, while concentrating on a problem. It's specific algorithm within acupuncture and meridian point tapping, where you tap on nine acupressure points (The Tapping Solution, n/d). EFT teaches that you can tap these specific acupressure points while you focus on the memories of the hurt and trauma from the abuse. With this, you will discover that you can access the memory without the anxiety, allowing the victim to let go of all the negative emotions associated with the trauma of the relationship.

How EFT Works

Often, when we are anxious and stressed, it is because of unrest and feeling threatened. This is common with victims of narcissistic abuse. When the body feels threatened, it switches to the "fight or flight" mode because of the activation of the amygdala. We see the physical manifestation of this through sweat, increased heart rate, muscles tensing up, etc. This is our body's reaction to the threat—which is helpful if we do need to confront a physical danger, but taxing on the body otherwise.

The issue, however, is that the brain has not evolved to distinguish between a life-threatening situation and a perceived threat. As a result, the trauma and aftermath of a relationship with a narcissist can trigger the same physical response our forefathers had when they faced a tiger.

You can calm the body by tapping the end points of the meridian. This sends a signal to the amygdala that you are not confronting a tiger. To make this more effective, we recommend doing the tapping while discussing or creating images of the stressful relationship and breakup. This way, the tapping alters the body's response to the images.

From the above, it is evident that you can use tapping as a tool to relax your mind when you feel overwhelmed by the trauma.

In employing tapping, we recommend that you ascribe a number to whatever you feel, be it physical or emotional. Let's assume it is a physical emotion, then you put a number to your feeling, on a scale from one to 10, with 10 being severely painful and one is barely feeling it. If it is emotions, consider how angry, distressed, or anxious (whatever the emotion) you feel on a scale from one to 10. If you are addressing some limiting belief like low self-esteem on a scale from one to 10, how do I value myself?

This is known as the subjective units of distress.

We recommend measuring your response since it can serve as a tool to know how you are progressing. Without this, people discard the feeling quickly once they feel better, without considering how they felt before. This is due to the rapid disconnection from the old feeling, which is expected since there was no measurement of said feeling.

As soon as you have your SUD level, start tapping and accompany it with a setup statement. The setup statement takes this format: "Even though I... (add the issue and a soothing statement)." For instance, "Even though I am anxious, I have complete control of my faculties," "Even though I do not feel confident, I have faith in my ability."

Whatever the result of the trauma, customize the statement and add a fact that can help counteract the negative emotions. With this, you can accept yourself and develop self-love. Many people have realized that tapping can help clear away past hurt, trauma, resentment, or other effects of abuse such that it does not hold you back.

Tapping helps balance your energy and expel negative emotions from the body. The natural balanced state of man, what we were born with, is that of joy and happiness. With tapping, you can eliminate tension and emotions blocking the natural balance until there is room for joy and happiness, rather than being held down by the trauma.

The human mind is like a garden. As long as there are weeds (negative emotions, pain from trauma and abuse, anxiety, etc.) you can't have a peaceful mind. This is why you need to get rid of these emotions for you to return your mind to a state of calmness, love, joy, and peace.

Yoga for Narcissist Abuse Recovery

When we talk about yoga, it is not about expensive outfits and equipment, or funny stretches and poses. Yoga can help victims of abuse or trauma experience relieve from symptoms like anxiety, stress, fear, feelings of inadequacy, etc. Direct and indirect exposure to trauma puts our thoughts in a state of captivity. As a result, the body reacts by activating the sympathetic nervous system, putting us in a constant state of fight or flight and, at times, it paralyzes us.

Trauma can be an assault to the balance of the body. This assault consumes the mind, body, and soul keeping it in a constant state of imbalance and negative conditioning.

With yoga, however, you can restructure the involuntary reaction of the sympathetic nervous system. In addition, it helps to bring back the balance by bringing about mindful, voluntary, and deliberate alignment of the body and breath. This helps get rid of trauma, whether physical or emotional, that is laden all over the body—the joints, the brain, connecting tissues, and the muscles.

While doing yoga, these various segments of the body are triggered and nurtured, which helps guide the body back to balance. Yoga presents a safe practice that is conditioned to the body of the survivor. As a result, they can safely process and engage, and sustain their sensation through the various phases of healing. Yoga creates an accessible and self-directed space which helps reintegrate the mind, body, and spirit. As victims explore everything yoga has to offer, sensation can flow through their body, allowing pain to dissipate.

Yoga is a practice that combines breath with a presence of mind. This brings peace, as well as a release of tension. Yoga is a physical practice that allows survivors to explore their emotions, sensations, feelings, etc., with curiosity. With this, you can develop a unique attitude with which you embrace all that happens with compassion.

Mirror Exposure Therapy

Mirror exposure therapy also helps treat negative self-image, reduce anxiety, and other damaging aftermath of breaking up with a narcissistic partner. It is a pretty effective strategy that helps you develop self-love and learn to accept yourself. Continuous exposure to criticism and abuse from a narcissist can deal a big blow to one's self-esteem. You will then find yourself doing things to please the narcissistic partner, even if it means changing who you are.

Rather than getting uncomfortable, tensed up and dissatisfied with who you are (due to the brainwashing from the narcissist), this therapy can help you accept who you are without shame. The aim of mirror exposure therapy is to suppress and eliminate the unconscious process that makes a reflection of the victim become an object of torture.

Prolonged exposure to narcissistic abuse does not only sap your self-esteem, it also make victims lose their identity. In addition to low self-esteem, their self-worth is punctured such that the victim does not attach any value to their personality. As a result, it is not uncommon for such people to regard themselves with disdain and failure. Failure in falling for an abusive partner and being so daft as to get carried away by the charms of such manipulator. These people feel so disgusted with themselves that beholding themselves in the mirror leads to disgust and probably reminders of when the abuser got physical.

Consider a healthy person, for instance—this person does not have any issue with the body's reflection in the mirror. They love themselves, accept their flaws, and do not feel disgusted at the sight of their reflection. Abused people are, however, turned off by flaws that are all in their head, which causes extreme pain and suffering.

Mirror exposure therapy is of tremendous help in this

kind of circumstance. Also, this therapy works best when combined with an effective management of the emotions and negative thoughts. In other words, for you to have tangible relief with this therapy, you need to handle this in two processes.

How Mirror Exposure Therapy Works

Many victims of abuse have shown significant improvement after going through mirror therapy. They had improved self-esteem with reduced cortisol levels. They also could accept who they are without taking responsibility for the battered relationship.

Significant improvement in patients going through mirror work is possible because of the pillars in which the process revolves.

Readjustment of Self-Interpretation: After a traumatic breakup, the victim might associate everything that goes wrong in their life with the breakup. This therapy helps terminate such prediction, while allowing the client have a healthy interpretation.

Attention Bias: Over time, the victim might attribute

the failure of the relationship to their own imperfections. Regret sets in and they wish they could be better and more tolerant. This therapy helps realign such thoughts with reality. Nothing is wrong with them, the relationship was just not meant to be.

Reduction of Anxiety and Fear: Problematic and negative emotions will surge during the breakup. Mirror work helps the patient develop a positive relationship with themselves such that depression, anxiety, and fear have no way to set in.

Without a doubt, this therapy is a terrific tool in bringing sanity to a victim of narcissistic abuse. All in all, it gives you the courage to accept yourself, be happy, shake off the negative emotions, and prepare yourself for what life has to offer.

Art Therapy

There will be various surges of distressing emotions upon ending a narcissistic relationship. It is not uncommon for people in this category to experience anxiety and symptoms of Post-Traumatic Stress Disorder. Art therapy has proven to be fairly effective in helping people heal from the emotional trauma caused by a narcissistic relationship.

For centuries, art therapy has been used as an effective tool for tackling all sorts of mental health issues. It can help everyone process a traumatic event such that healing will be swift.

The effect of trauma in the body is overwhelming. Trauma causes both physical and emotional reactions in the victim. It is common for victims to experience disturbing flashbacks, sleep disturbances, panic and anxiety, anger, depression, and guilt. As a result, the person's normal functioning in day-to-day activities might be impaired. Art therapy is an effective treatment that can help restore sanity.

Traumatic experiences and memories from narcissistic abuse exist in our bodies and minds in state-specific form. In other words, they exist in the body the same way when the event happened, typically giving the same visual, emotional, and physiological experience. As a result of this, to recover from PTSD arising from narcissistic abuse, victims must be willing to work through such unprocessed memories until they stop triggering disturbing symptoms.

PTSD occurs through emotions, memories, and the body. This is why talk therapy and CBT alone might not be able to address it. This is where art therapy comes in.

What is Art Therapy?

Art is a means of expression, like writing or speaking, with which you can communicate things that would otherwise be diluted. However, one might wonder at the role of art and art therapy in helping a trauma victim?

There are times victims of trauma abuse may feel lost. It could be difficult for them to find the right words to express their emotions. This is where art therapy comes in, as a rescue to trauma victim when they feel stuck. Therefore, with art therapy, clients can:

- Express complex emotions like rage, sadness, grief, etc, without uttering a word

- Get creative by tapping into the right side of the brain

- Use various mediums to express themselves and process their emotions (like paint, pencil, marker, color, photography, collage, etc.)

People can deal with stress and anxiety, improve their self-esteem, and develop insights that can be a ticket to a more fulfilling life with art therapy. The therapy is done under the guidance of the art therapist (usually an artist). Either the therapist or the client can choose the medium of expression. However, the medium of art expression chosen should be what appeals to the client.

How Art Therapy Helps Victims

Art therapy employs various forms of art to address mental health issues and help victims of abuse or trauma. It can be combined with a talk therapy, but it is also effective as a stand-alone therapy. The sole aim is not to come up with an artwork. Rather, art therapy helps foster self-expression and self-awareness. When clients color, paint, or express themselves through any other means, it creates a safe and conducive medium to process a painful event from the past. With coloring, for instance, client can engage various parts of their brain which helps them deal with the trauma differently.

In art therapy, clients express feelings and thoughts

about trauma by making an illustration of their reaction and talking about it. With art, clients can develop coping skills by photographing pleasant and soothing objects.

Art therapy is very effective since talk therapy might not encompass a person's whole experience. This is because there are times words fail to express what someone is going through. With art, you can access experience, information, and probably emotions that you might not get to through words.

Healing and recovery after narcissistic abuse also has to do with reclaiming the safety of your body, emotions, and senses. Prolonged exposure to narcissistic abuse can make victims feel disconnected from their body. This is due to the constant threat from their abuser which leads to feeling of unsafe, and constant fear during the period of the abuse. To fully recover from such abuse, however, victims need to develop new relationships with their bodies. Victims need to be aware of the body's sensations, as well as the mode of interaction of their body with the world around them. This is why self-awareness is critical to healing.

Art work is effective for body work because victims can manipulate artwork outside themselves. Victims can express difficult pieces of their traumatic event through various means. This enables them to access their physical experience, which helps create a realization that their body is a safe place.

Sample Art Therapy Exercise for Healing

Emotions

You can deal with emotions like sadness, grief, and anger through the following art therapy exercises:

I. **Draw your heart:** Draw a heart—your heart—and input all your feelings with symbols and illustrations.

II. **Line art:** This is one of the simplest and most basic aspects of art which can help express a lot of emotions. With line art, you can reveal how you feel.

III. **Make a postcard you will never send:** Are you still mad and upset with the narcissist? Design a postcard that shows just how you feel. You shouldn't actually send this, though.

IV. **Paint a mountain and a valley**: The mountain

stands for a time you were happy, probably prior to the relationship. And the valley, a time you were sad. Draw this and add whatever reflects how you feel.

Relaxation

Art therapy can help you relax. The following exercises can have a calming effect on your nerves, amidst all the surge of emotions after the separation:

I.   **Use colors that calm you:** Choose any color that appeals to you and make a drawing or a painting.

II. **Draw with your eyes closed:** When you can't see what you are drawing, it encourages intuition, sensitivity, and touch.

III. **Employ a color book**: Colors are associated with varieties of emotions. Select various paint chips to paint, collage, and glue until you have a colorful masterpiece.

Trauma and Loss

At times, to truly heal, you need to come face to face with unpleasant things in your life. With this, you can develop the courage to surmount them.

I.   **Draw a place where you feel safe:** Tap into your imagination to find where you feel relaxed, amidst the hurt, woes, and surge of emotions overwhelming you.

II.   **Collage away your worries:** By cutting, tearing, shredding, and layering, you can toss your worries and fears away.

III. **Make a momentary art:** Many cultures practice sand painting for healing purpose. Using sand on canvas, you can create patterns that appeal to you.

IV.   **Make a drawing of something that scares you:** What is that thing about the trauma that keeps you up at night? That sends your heart racing? You can express this fear via drawing and, hopefully, you can face it.

On a final note, with art therapy, you can address the trauma of the abuse and its effect in your entire being: the body, soul, and spirit. You can work through PTSD by employing art, which can help reduce the blow of the trauma.

Chakra Balancing

Energy healing is a deep practice that triggers the energy system hidden in the body. This helps get rid of blockages, keeps the mind at peace, and brings serenity to your spirit. Breaking through these energy blocks activates the body's ability to heal itself. It is a holistic healing method that encompasses the spirit, soul, and body.

Energy healing employed by chakra healing has its basis in science and ancient principles. Chakra has been proven to heal the deepest of wounds, and trauma that might arise from any traumatic experience. To understand how to heal with chakra, the concept of energy body is vital.

At its most basic, the human body is made of energy. By energy body, we mean a system that conveys life force around and through us. This life force energy connects us to the earth, to one another, and to the divine. There is this thing in you that knows when someone is toxic, when their energy feels good, and when there is tranquility in their aura.

The energy body has two major components: the aura and chakra systems.

The Aura

The aura is like an electric energy field coming from your body in bubbles. It is like energy layers that come from your personal chakras. It is seen as colors, based on the vibrations they give.

The body energy is in a constant state of change, based on the physical and emotional health. People can feel their energy change which serves two critical purposes: protection and information exchange.

The Aura and Protection

The aura is like a barrier of energy that stands between you and the environment. A healthy aura provides a sense of security, keeping you from the energy of others emanating around you. Your boundary is clear, enabling you tell the difference between your emotions and needs from those of others.

With an unhealthy aura, on the other hand, you are anxious, fearful, depressed, etc. Your boundary is poor, so the energy of everyone around seems to come down heavily on you. As a result, their emotions and issues become yours.

The aura, however, is vital to emotional health. This is because part of the basic needs of humans are safety and acceptance, which keep us going. With a strong aura, there is that confidence that you are safe and protected, free to face the world and all it throws at you.

The Aura and Information Exchange

The aura also serves as a field of information where you exchange data with people you meet. Even if you don't know it, this exchange takes place with everyone you encounter.

Many people do not realize this, but if you reflect back, I am sure you will realize some interactions in which you knew things about another person. You know when something just does not feel right. We have met people at times and we feel drawn to them, like we already knew them for ages. We have also met people and felt uncomfortable or scared around them. How did you know this? You 'read' the person's aura with yours. This is what others call vibe, or vibration.

In general, everyone gives an unconscious reaction to information coming from their aura. However, the goal is to equip you such that you are conscious of it. This way, you can tap its healing power and use it to heal yourself, physically and emotionally. Bear in mind that trauma is stored both in the cellular level of the physical body and the energy body. This is why, for you to truly heal and recover from the narcissistic abuse, you need to let go of trauma from these places.

The Chakras

There are various energy centers in the body that represents areas of emotional, spiritual, and physical functioning. The body has seven main chakras, which are linked to each other through the energy channels that run through the body. This book will discuss the essential ones for the sake of recovery after a traumatic breakup.

In the body, there is a constant recycling of energetic breath. While new energy comes in, old ones are expelled. With your breath, you can transport energy through your body. The breath serves as a bridge between what we are feeling and what we want to feel.

Root Chakra

The foundation of the energy body is the root chakra. It

is located at the center of the body, in the base of the spine, and passes through the leg to the sole of the feet. When viewed, it is red in color.

It is responsible for safety, stability, and survival in your life. The balance of the root chakra creates a strong sense of security and confidence. You feel grounded with the audacity to take risks and enjoy all life throws at you. An imbalanced root chakra makes one afraid, anxious, fearful, etc. Restoring your root chakra is vital to combating anxiety and gets rid of the need to fight for survival.

Sacral Chakra

Located just below your belly button is the sacral chakra. This is the center of emotional expression, core beliefs, and creativity. A balanced sacral chakra will bring joy and a sense of fulfillment. It is usually seen as orange.

A balanced sacral chakra makes you confident in your skin. You feel empowered to handle everything life throws at you. You should aim to balance the sacral chakra after leaving an abusive relationship. This is because an unbalanced sacral chakra makes you question your self-worth, besides becoming judgmental.

Solar Plexus Chakra

Located at the base of your sternum, this is usually yellow in color. It controls will, self-esteem, and your power. Being your powerhouse, it controls how you influence the world around you. A balanced solar plexus chakra makes you feel strong, confident, and able to go after what you want.

Many victims of narcissistic abuse have an unbalanced solar plexus chakra. When it is out of balance, you are easily controlled by others, you do not know what you really want, and get easily irritated. Balancing this chakra can help you gain the freedom you want. It helps you move ahead, with new hope and faith in yourself to flourish in a new relationship.

Heart Chakra

Located at the center of the chest is the heart chakra. This is where love and all the relationships you will have in life are located, even your relationship with yourself. Represented by the color green, a balanced heart chakra helps bring balance between receiving and giving.

With a balanced heart chakra, you will have a stable and supportive relationship. You can love and feel worthy to receive love. Balancing the heart chakra is essential to healing—and an unbalanced heart chakra, on the other hand, makes you give excessively since you have poor boundaries. This should be one of your aims after ending a narcissistic relationship. It makes you whole and prepares you for the next relationship.

Throat Chakra

Located in the hollow of your throat is the throat chakra. It is the center of communication as it helps with self-validation and active listening. A balanced throat chakra helps you express yourself and your feelings without fear. It is also the key to hearing what others have to say.

Many victims of narcissistic abuse have their throat chakra out of balance. An unbalanced throat chakra makes you put the needs of others above your own. You do not get to express yourself well, which means you may beholding back your emotions and needs. A balanced throat chakra will stop making you see yourself as a victim of narcissistic abuse. Rather, you see this as a step in the journey to where you are meant to be.

It is evident that chakra balancing is one of the keys to

getting your life in order after the trauma of a narcissistic relationship. There are resources online that can guide you on specific practices to help balance your chakra. Chakra balance is a holistic approach to recovery that can help transform and restore your health, while preparing you for your next relationship.

Chapter 6: Pillars of Recovery After Narcissistic Abuse

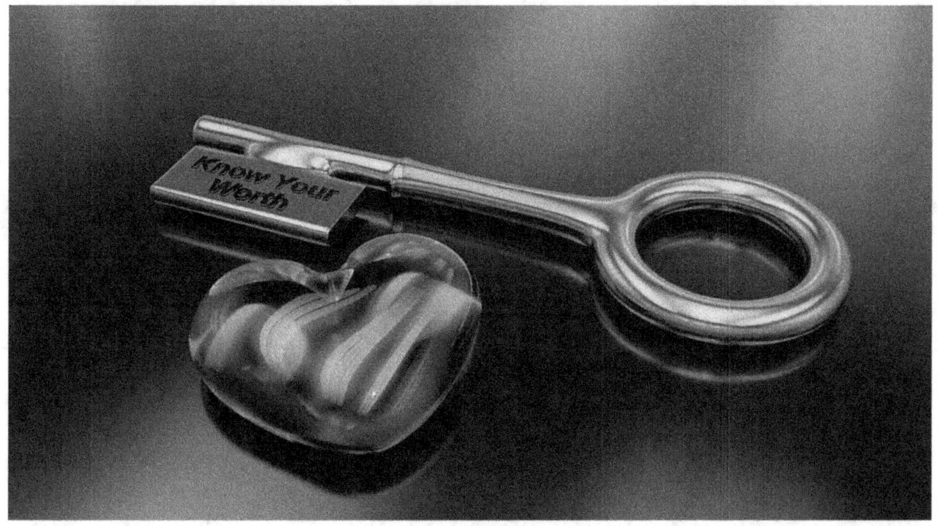

We recommend various strategies for survival. Most trauma recovery tips involve going to a therapist and getting in touch with a guide. This chapter, however, focuses on what you can do for yourself from the comfort of your home. Even if you lack the willpower and motivation to go out and get help, you can help yourself right where you are.

The following explains significant aspects of your life you can work on, on your own.

Self-Esteem

Self-esteem has to do with having confidence in yourself and your abilities. It has to do with how you see yourself and the effect your immediate environment has on you.

When your self-esteem becomes battered, it shows through self-sabotage and self-destruction. When your self-esteem is low, you find yourself doing things to destroy your own opportunities. You stop trying or even give up immediately after starting.

After the narcissistic abuse, you develop self-hatred, which affects how you relate to yourself. You might even resort to substance abuse, excessive spending, etc. You lose interest in things and have no desire to make any effort, since your last relationship was filled with you trying to fix things, fix that person, without positive results.

Building your self-esteem involves putting yourself back in the game. It involves developing the willpower to launch yourself out all over again. However, you should start small. We are talking about baby steps, little things that will give you a sense of accomplishment. It can be as simple as taking care of yourself, washing the dishes that have been piling up, going to the movies, giving yourself a treat, etc.

Self-Worth

When we talk about self-worth, we mean how much you value and respect yourself. That is, knowing yourself and what you are worth.

After narcissistic abuse, it is common to be filled with shame and a sense of unworthiness. This is when the voices in your head tell you "you are not good enough." Being in a narcissistic relationship has a way of sapping your self-worth—in a bid to save your relationship with this person, you compromise on some of your values.

Over time, you will be afraid of speaking up for yourself. You might find it difficult to open up to those that will help you. Even if people do something bad, you will not be able to express yourself. Yet, deep down, you are castigating and confronting yourself. Absence of self-worth also manifest in the lack of interest in taking care of yourself and meeting your needs.

To build your self-worth, you need to be courageous. In

other words, you have got to take risks and start small. You might be fearful but, deep down, you want that thing. You need to take steps to go after what you want. It could be about going out more, showing up at the party, meeting new people. It could even be putting yourself out there and dating again after leaving the abusive relationship.

Another way to boost your self-worth is to know what your values are, and live by them. After this, you need protection in the form of boundaries and standards. It does not stop here—you also need the willpower to defend them, once pushed. Bear in mind that your last relationship was filled with your boundaries being pushed anyhow, without much effort from you to check in.

Self-Trust

This involves knowing and believing in yourself. Lack of self-trust will show up as doubt and fear. This is the fear that cripples your creativity, and stops you from taking risks and connecting with others.

When you lack self-trust, you will second-guess yourself. In other words, no matter how strong and beautiful the idea you have, you lack confidence in yourself to say or do it. You have beaten yourself up so much for falling in love and starting a relationship with a jerk. This battered your confidence and you lack trust in your ability to make other positive decisions.

Lack of self-trust also shows up in simple day-to day-decisions you need to make. You might be confused on the clothes to pick for an outing, it could be indecision about a brand of margarine, etc. This could be due to walking on eggshells around your former abusive partner. While in that relationship, you never knew the next thing you might do to set him off. Hence, even after leaving them, you find yourself still stuck in the circle of indecision.

What indecision does is to keep you stuck, with a sense of paralysis. The ability to commit to something is not there. You might lack the power to handle all life throws at you, which will make you insecure.

To rebuild your self-trust, you need to connect with and listen to your intuition. In other words, listen to your body and your feelings about something, someone, an idea, and a situation. On knowing this, you will let it come to focus in your body. Acting on your intuition can help rebuild trust in yourself. You will lose when you fail to listen to your intuition, which will batter your self-esteem all the more, since you lack the willpower to do what you want.

To rebuild your self-trust, integrity must guide your actions. This is where your values coincide with your actions. When you have complete faith in yourself, it will rebuild your sense of trust since you are capable of setting boundaries that will protect you. Not only that, your actions will be in alignment with what you value.

Self-Love

When you love yourself, you will care and nurture yourself. You will accept yourself with your flaws and treat yourself right.

Without self-love, however, you will be judgmental and deny yourself a lot of things. This also manifests in you doing things to please other people. This is not surprising, as your broken relationship was filled with you trying to please your abusive partner. Even after the relationship, you may find yourself sacrificing your needs for those of others. You let them trample on you in a bid to keep the connection or relationship.

What are the kind of things you tell yourself? We all have this constant conversation going on in our head. You might condemn yourself or put yourself down constantly through the voices in your head. When you lack self-love, you treat yourself poorly, you do not value yourself enough to take care of yourself. This could manifest in mundane things like overeating or under-eating, consuming excessive junk foods or alcohol, or indulging in other addictions.

Lack of self-love could also manifest in the form of compromising what you need to do for the needs of others. Bear in mind that compromising in this sense might not be a big deal, if it is only minute things. However, when it comes to compromising your integrity, peace, health, well-being, or sanity, you need to be mindful.

We all make mistakes at times. With poor self-love, we end up talking down or even abusing ourselves, saying things like, "dumbass," or "how could I have been so stupid?" etc. Even after the breakup, you end up castigating yourself for falling to the tactics of the abuser, hating yourself in the process.

To develop self-love, you need to start caring for yourself. This is an all-round care that encompasses the physical, mental, emotional, and spiritual health.

You can develop self-love by taking steps to address things about yourself that you can adjust. This should be what you have control over. For the things that you cannot change, like your height or skin color, you have to accept them. This is where self-acceptance comes in. Work on silencing these negative voices. You could have unconsciously internalized the criticism and condemnation of the narcissist. The narcissist abused and condemned you such that you felt guilty for your flaws, leading to self-condemnation and guilt in the process.

By loving yourself, you can take the necessary steps to change the things you can, and begin to work on accepting yourself.

Self-Kindness and Understanding

This is an important aspect of ending a relationship with a narcissist. You need to be kind to yourself in the process.

Reflect on the relationship you just ended. You will break down many times. You will second-guess yourself, leading to self-doubt with a loss of faith in yourself and your ability to function without your abusive partner.

The key here is to recognize and accept that you deserve more. You have inner strength that has been suppressed due to constant and excessive interaction with the narcissist. All you need to do is bring out this strength once again.

Bear in mind that this will take time—more time than is needed to heal from a healthy relationship. This is why you need to be kind to yourself and accept that your healing will not come in a single day. Self-kindness is a powerful virtue that will get you through the ordeal of the breakup. Give yourself a treat, go and have a night out with the girls. Do this until it becomes part of you. You deserve better!

In Summary

We have shed light on five vital pillars that are critically affected and battered due to a prolonged relationship with a narcissist. As a result, if you want your recovery to be successful, you need to prioritize working on these pillars. No matter how much relationship with your ex has battered your self-esteem and made you question your relevance, you *can* get your life in order again.

The good news is that you can take steps today, without seeing a therapist or an external party, to help you work on these virtues. However, if you find that you are struggling, be sure to get help to assist you get back on your feet.

Conclusion

Breaking up is hard, but breaking up with a narcissist is even harder. This is due to the physical, psychological, and emotional damage the relationship has on the victim. The good news, however, is that you can recover. You can get your life in order such that getting back out there does not seem like a tedious task.

Maybe you feel worthless, drained, and unlike yourself after the relationship—but you can get help. It might even seem like the end of your life and existence; however, it is not. You can rise up again and get back on your feet.

Imprinted in the pages of this book are tested and proven tips that will give a complete transformation of your physical, emotional, psychological, and mental health. It might take time, but you will heal. Be sure to follow the tactics and steps recommended in this manual. Do not beat yourself up if the improvements do not come at a rapid speed. All the havoc caused by the narcissist did not happen in a day, hence it will take time to heal. As a result, you need to be patient with yourself. Celebrate the gradual improvement and anticipate more to come.

We have provided many practical steps that can help get you back on your feet. In other words, this is not about knowledge alone. You have got to read it and take the recommended steps. This way, you can stop beating yourself up and shake off the phobia of relationships that the narcissist caused you.

Healing and recovery is possible after narcissistic abuse. You can pick yourself up and put yourself out there for a better and more meaningful relationship.